DR. BRIAI

MW00624763

(UN)RESOLVED

HARNESSING YOUR MOVEMENT STORY
TO END CHRONIC PAIN

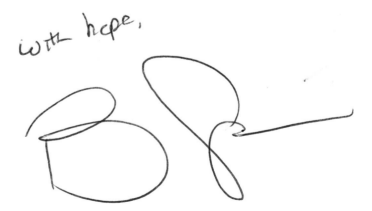

with hope,

Praise for Brian Yee's *(Un)Resolved*

"Brian Yee is the thinking person's physical therapist. Instead of treating the injury in front of him, he treats the entire person. He will change the way you think about your body, and may very well help you discover the reason you are in pain — and what you need to do, holistically, to leave that pain behind."

- Cathryn Jakobson Ramin, author of *Crooked: Outwitting the Back Pain Industry and Getting on the Road to Recovery*

"Brian is a trusted practitioner and a wise friend. His message is so hopeful and helpful in re-writing the oppressive story of chronic pain. What a timely and timeless resource to bring much-longed-for healing to so many!"

- Jay & Katherine Wolf, co-authors of *Hope Heals* and *Suffer Strong*

"This book that Dr. Brian Yee has written is great because it does what is needed to help people solve their pain: meet the sufferer where they are and guide them to a better place. Solving long-term pain is a process; it involves walking along a path of learning and change. Dr. Yee paves the way so the person can explore their uniqueness, learn many strategies, and morph into someone who can control their own pain."

- Michael Shacklock, Founder of Neurodynamic Solutions

"This book will help so many people understand that there's still hope and solutions for their pain—even if they have had it for a long time. Dr. Brian Yee masterfully explains all of the factors that make up a person's pain experience. This will help people understand how to recognize the contributing elements and signs of their own pain story and how to seek the appropriate help from a full body approach."

- Tracy Sher, Founder of Pelvic Guru

"Looking back at my career, there was a time where, I certainly didn't know at the time, I learned the most about pain and pain science. Pain is so contextual and based on beliefs and mental conditioning, but the reality is those constructs are all still based in physiology. They can be explained. They can be measured. They can be manipulated. Dr. Yee's text here will explain what I saw before pain science burgeoned and became popular. He explains the links between perception and hard physiology in a well-written illustrative storyboard. I expect all will enjoy and be enlightened."

- Charlie Weingroff, Former Strength and Conditioning Coach, Philadelphia 76ers, NBA | Former Lead Physical Therapist, United States Marine Corps Special Operations Command

This book is dedicated to my amazing wife, Eileen, who spurred me on to complete this book.

© 2022 Brian Yee

All rights reserved. No part of this book may be reproduced in any form or by any electronic or mechanical means, including information storage and retrieval systems, without permission in writing from the author and illustrator, except in the case of brief quotations in the context of critical articles or reviews.

ISBN 978-1-7379509-0-5 (paperback)
ISBN 978-1-7379509-1-2 (eBook)

Cover design and interior layout by Aaxel Author Services & Noah Adam Paperman

This book is designed for educational purposes only. You should not rely on this information as a substitute for, nor does it replace, professional medical advice, diagnosis, or treatment. If you have any concerns or questions about your health, you should always consult with a physician or other health-care professional. Do not disregard, avoid or delay obtaining medical or health related advice from your health-care professional because of something you may have read in this book. The use of any information provided in this book is solely at your own risk.

Table of Contents

Introduction:

Pain and the Role of Physical Therapy

What comes to mind when you think of physical therapy? For most people, it's often tied to pain, surgery, or an injury. You might think it's only something you need after a specific incident, like a sprained ankle or a nagging muscle. In this case, physical therapy is probably something you only consider when you're referred by your primary care doctor. You see a physical therapist, receive heat or electrical treatment, get a list of recommended exercises, and, with any luck, do them until you feel better. That's it, right?

Not quite. In reality, physical therapy can—and in most cases should—come well before you're faced with an injury, surgery, or ongoing pain. A well-trained physical therapist will spend more time getting to know you and pinpointing the real root of your concerns. This kind of approach is designed to not only relieve your existing pain, but also to help prevent pain or injury in the future. This way a physical therapist can teach you how to use your body the most effective way possible.

But why would anyone seek physical therapy without a referral? Well, maybe you're experiencing what seems to be never-ending pain. Or maybe you know someone who is. Maybe at this point you (or they) have already been to a primary care physician, seen a specialist, or tried a number of medications and treatments without any improvement. Or maybe the pain went away for a while only to return. Maybe now you want to take a more involved, proactive approach to taking care of yourself.

If so, let me be the first to welcome and congratulate you for starting the journey toward resolving your pain. This is a path of discovery, empowerment, and growth. It can be challenging at times, but in the end, you'll be able to reclaim your body and enjoy activities you may have left behind. And I'm here to help you find your way.

Who am I? My name is Brian Yee, and I'm a Doctor of Physical Therapy, a Board-Certified Orthopedic Clinical Specialist (OCS), and Fellow of the American Academy of Orthopaedic Manual Physical Therapists (AAOMPT). My practice is founded upon exploring every possible, seemingly unrelated cause that leads to pain—no matter what kind. And although I've been practicing for twenty years, in some ways the health of others has always had a role in my life.

It all started with my dad. Ever since I was young, he practiced as a pharmacist in his own small, family-run business with a philosophy based on customer service and personal touch. What does that mean exactly? It means he took a deliberately slow and personalized approach to dealing with his patients. When people came into his pharmacy, he took extra time to get to know them, their family members, and all the details about their lives.

Eventually his patients came to see him as more than just another medical professional delivering a service—they saw him as a member of their family. And instead of blindly filling prescription after prescription, my father treated his customers like real people with real hopes and dreams. Most importantly, he helped his patients every day by providing camaraderie, friendship, and compassion as well as medication.

Needless to say, my father's philosophy greatly influenced my life. As I got older, I saw a stark contrast between his approach and some of the more common methods that are often rushed and impersonal. To me, it seemed simply impossible that anyone could understand another person's injury or pain from one brief conversation, and my interest in physical therapy was born of a desire to adopt my father's model and help people truly heal.

After finishing graduate studies in Physical Therapy at Northwestern University, I realized I was just getting started. I wanted to know more, so I completed an advanced degree in Physiotherapy at the University of Queensland in Australia, where they house a world-class physiotherapy program.

During my time in Australia, I got to participate in extensive research and training around chronic pain rehabilitation. Under the supervision of senior therapists, I began to treat patients with unresolved pain. In every instance, my mentors made sure I understood who the patient was, what could be causing their pain, and what the best method of treatment would be for them as a unique individual.

In a nutshell, the program made me think about my every interaction with a patient. It taught me to take a moment to be humble and ask myself to be a better clinician before probing the patient. Taking a deductive approach allows the patient to tell their story and answer questions about their physical structure as well as their mental, spiritual, and social environments. This way, we can shed light on when and why the pain started, what may have caused it, and what other medical conditions might be at the root of the problem—all without ever touching the patient.

Like my father's approach, this model is much different than today's typical healthcare experience. Where most people wait at length only to receive a superficial solution, I saw an opportunity to create a practice that treats patients with dedicated and uninterrupted time. I use that time to truly get to know the person behind the chronic pain, recurring injury, or sports performance goal.

Don't misunderstand me: there's a time and place for many different types of medical treatments, and that's exactly why I've taken a different approach. I don't believe in treating symptoms with one-size-fits-all medications or exercises; I believe in meeting a person where they are and providing them with the tools they need to get well and stay well.

Perhaps one of my greatest strengths as a physical therapist lies in my ability to share my knowledge of the human body and how it all works together. Because when you know more, you can better understand how pain works, why it occurs, what changes it causes in your body, and how it can affect the way you move every day.

But the other value I always want to add is using compassion as a tool to peer behind someone's pain complaints and determine what really drives that person's core identity and purpose. I believe that if I know what moves someone intrinsically, and how he or she ultimately desires to live, I can more accurately correlate who a person is with why they are in chronic pain. I've found that until you take the time to understand the spiritual and aspirational components of a person in chronic pain you will struggle to get to the bottom of their pain.

It's why I started Motion Stability, Atlanta's leading center for the diagnosis and treatment of unresolved pain, movement, and performance rehabilitation. It's also the reason I wanted to write this book. What I can offer you is a chance to step away from the frustration of dealing with specific, isolated pain and see the greater, more complex story behind its cause.

Unfortunately, I can't give you a list of ten simple exercises to end back pain for good. And although I cannot provide treatment within these chapters, I can provide information about the reasons pain exists and encourage you to consider a different approach to finding relief.

At the end of the day, this book is designed to help you find strategies that overthrow the feeling of hopelessness and frustration about your pain, so you can make changes to improve your life and advocate for your body. Ultimately, my goal is to restore your hope for a life without pain.

To make our journey as easy as possible, I've divided the book into two parts, each with three distinct sections. In Part One, the first section is intended to share the importance of getting a broader perspective of your pain. The second section is set up to help you understand your pain narrative, and it includes practical steps to guide you as you put your pain into the context of who you are. The last section in Part One is intended to help you understand what happens within your body when pain occurs.

In Part Two, the first section will explore how your body is designed and how it physically functions. We'll cover what happens to your body after injury or pain occurs, what we call remnant changes, and how these changes affect the way your body works. The second section ties it all together by combining and integrating your narrative and your body's design. And finally, the third section will provide practical steps for you to take moving forward because, unfortunately, this book alone will not be able to fix your pain.

Instead, my goal is to give you the right perspective so you can start your journey toward resolving your pain the correct way. You'll find a handful of real-life cases to help guide your understanding throughout the book, as well as a number of underlined words for which you can find corresponding definitions in the glossary at the end.

Ultimately, my goal is to teach you everything you need to know to have a better understanding of your own pain experience. I'll help you learn how to ask the right questions, figure out why your pain is occurring, find caring practitioners, seek proper treatment, and, finally, get back to living.

PART ONE

Discovering the Roots of Your
Pain

Section 1.1:

Dealing with Pain in Today's Healthcare

Here you are: You finally decided to pick up this book because you or a loved one is experiencing some sort of bodily pain that has been ongoing, nagging, or flat-out frustrating. Perhaps it has just begun or perhaps it has already consumed a majority of your life. At minimum, it has significantly altered the way you move and impacted your lifestyle or the life you want to live—and you've finally had enough. And even though you have sought out medical examination and have been ruled out of any pathology that is life-threatening, you might find yourself saying things like, "Why is my pain still here?" Or, "Why can no one figure out why it is happening?" Or, "There has to be a way out of this. I can't live in pain like this the rest of my life." So with some toggling combination of fear, frustration, and hope you've decided you're willing to go all in to get to the bottom of what's happening in your body, what's causing your pain, and how you can get yourself feeling better.

Because, if you're reading this, I'm willing to bet you're not the type of person who simply sits around doing nothing about your pain. My guess is you've been highly proactive in seeking medical attention, both through traditional and Western medicine as well as alternative or holistic means. In each case, every practitioner or specialist may have given you some sound reasoning about your diagnosis. They likely recommended a treatment that gave you short-term relief, provided no relief at all, or, worse, aggravated your pain.

Through it all, the most frustrating thing is that no one seems to fully understand what's happening with you. Maybe you feel like each specialist threw a dart at the problem and hit a specific part of the issue, but no one has been able to put everything together well enough to make sense of the madness you're experiencing in your own body. Whether you suffer from sciatica, back or neck pain, a sharp pain in your hip when you run, or shoulder pain when you lift something, there is often more to the story than what any specialist can see in a single visit.

Rather than call your pain chronic, which I believe promotes a fatalist mentality that suggests you'll never get better, I refer to the type of pain you're experiencing as *unresolved*. From my perspective, calling it unresolved pain indicates that there is still a solution out there for you, you just need the right approach to find it.

Diane's Story

Diane came into my clinic after she was referred by an orthopedic surgeon. Initially, Diane saw the surgeon because she was seeking an opinion about revising a surgery she had had on her left knee six years earlier. Unfortunately, the first surgery she had didn't make her knee feel better. Instead her knee pain became worse and she developed sensations of burning and numbness near her knee and down her leg.

As the symptoms worsened and the nerve-related sensations arose, Diane followed the recommendation of her knee surgeon to seek the care of a spine surgeon. Because Diane was experiencing nerve-related symptoms down her leg, and a Magnetic Resonance Imaging (MRI) showed two herniated discs in her lower back, the spine surgeon recommended Diane have back surgery. This surgery was intended to alleviate pressure from the herniated discs that were pressing on her nerves, which the surgeon assumed was causing the burning sensation in her left leg.

Trusting that her doctors knew best, Diane agreed to have a two-level lumbar (lower back) vertebrae surgery in order to remove the herniated discs completely. Her hope was that this procedure would resolve the numbness and burning, as well as her knee pain, once and for all. But the nerve symptoms in her leg didn't improve. In fact, they became more aggravated after the back surgery, and the pain in her left knee still lingered. To make matters worse, the increased aggravation in her back made it harder for her to sit, bend, or stand, and she struggled to live a normal life.

With both the knee surgeon and the spine surgeon baffled as to why Diane was not improving, her frustration led her back to her own intuition. She couldn't help but wonder whether her original knee surgery had been done correctly or whether having another knee surgery would fix the problem. She wanted another opinion, so she used online reviews to find another orthopedic surgeon. When the second orthopedic surgeon examined Diane, he determined there was nothing structurally wrong with her knee and instead recommended she come see me.

At first glance, the way Diane stood looked off-kilter. She leaned noticeably to the right, like the Leaning Tower of Pisa. It's possible the other doctors saw these things, too, but as a physical therapist, I have been trained to observe the human body with an understanding of certain norms or ideals about how the body should look and how it should move. So, when a body does not look as it should, it starts a deductive process in my mind that's designed to determine what may be causing the abnormalities.

In Diane's case, the fact that she leaned to the right gave me enough information to make some conclusions about why her left knee hurt in the first place, why the back surgery did not help, and why she had developed ongoing nerve symptoms down her left leg.

Further examination revealed that Diane's left leg was physically longer than her right leg. In physical therapy, we call this a *structural leg-length discrepancy*. What happens is that the longer leg created a stilt-like or pole-like effect on her left side and, as a result, she was literally being pushed over to the right. Amazingly, her body constantly tried to adapt to her longer leg over the course of her life. As a result, her longer left leg placed more extraneous forces on her left knee than her right, causing it to wear down faster and resulting in her knee pain. These additional forces also placed more stress on the left side of her back causing her nerve symptoms in her left leg to become more irritated as well.

When I pointed out the way Diane stood and walked, she was so astonished she said, "No one has ever taken the time to look at me and see these things, including myself!" And even though she didn't fully understand what was happening in her body just yet, she could tell that the way she leaned and the way she put more weight on her left leg simply could not be a good thing.

While leg-length discrepancies are rare, I mentioned this case because most people do not realize how strategically our bodies are designed. More importantly, they don't realize how hard our bodies will work to keep moving forward and accomplish the tasks, movements, or athletic activities we aim to achieve. As it does, it will also do whatever it can to be as efficient, symmetrical, and level as possible; however, at the expense of doing so, it sometimes puts more stress on certain joints, muscles, ligaments, and discs in our spine. If our bodies are not able to handle such stresses, eventually these things can wear out, tear, strain, or cause pain. This is why we begin to feel the pain we do when we overdo it.

The problem is that once we feel pain in our knee, our shoulder, or our back, we automatically assume we need to fix the spot where it hurts instead of looking at the entire body and how its parts work together.

This is what happens to people like Diane. All she knew was her left knee hurt, and because that's what she complained about, that's all the doctor looked at. So, she had a surgery to correct it, and although surgery works for some people, for Diane it didn't solve the problem because there were other significant reasons that caused her left knee to be out of sorts. By focusing on her knee and not the real reason behind the pain, she actually had worse symptoms as a result of the surgery that was intended to heal her.

The Overspecialization of the Healthcare System

So, what went wrong? Well, imagine a cartoon that depicts a patient standing in front of a doctor because their knee hurts, and the doctor is leaning in so close to look at the patient's knee that their nose is nearly touching it. By being so close to the knee, however, the doctor cannot see that the patient is leaning all the way over to one side because the leg that hurts is substantially longer than the other. Rather than seeing that disparity, the physician is so focused on going back and forth between the knee, the X-rays, and the MRI scans that they cannot see anything else; they can only confirm what they can see is wrong with the knee.

Though this is an exaggerated example of a physician missing the point, it symbolizes the nature in which our healthcare system operates and it's representative of what Diane, and patients like her, often experience. In this sense, the problem is that the physician has taken an overly myopic approach to their examination to see their patient's entire story.

My experience has led me to believe that we live in an era of specialization, and it has caused us to lose our ability to see the big picture first. I don't mean to criticize the medical system, but what happens is that we as medical professionals, myself included, pursue opportunities in our healthcare training that focus specifically on the things in which we want to develop our expertise. Like a sports orthopedic surgeon who only repairs ligament tears in the knee, or a certified hand therapist who only treats injuries to the elbow, wrist, or hand.

Our specialization is driven in part by the vast opportunities we now have for training, mentorship, and fellowships, as well as the opportunities within our society to pursue our dreams and our specialties. It is also driven in part by the market. In most cases, a patient is not going to choose a general physician to perform their knee-replacement surgery. They are more likely to opt for a surgeon who has completed 2,000 knee replacements, is considered the industry leader, has been published in highly credible medical journals, and is at the forefront of developing new technologies in their field. I would not even blame the patient, because it seems logical and wise to have someone with vast experience and expertise perform the surgery.

However, the danger in this era of uber-specialization is that, as with Diane, specialists have become so specialized that when a patient comes in to see them, it is very easy to only see the patient through a narrow lens. At times it can cause the specialist to lose sight of the context around what might be happening.

In clinical terminology, this is known as *confirmation bias*. It is the notion that we are inclined to interpret new information as confirmation of our existing theories, and our myopic vision to confirm what we see through our narrow, specialist perspective means we may find ourselves blindsided by the truth. The advantage to specialization is when the patient's problem does fit within the confines of our specialty, the results are above and beyond successful.

These are the pros and cons to being laser-focused. In many cases, putting all your attention toward one task, one project, or one thing can be very productive, and many times we are not laser-focused enough to get the job done; however, if you stay too dialed into the project you are focused on, as you expand your tunnel vision, you may realize there are things you sacrificed or disregarded in order to stay focused on your target.

This is what Diane, and many patients dealing with unresolved pain, experienced. The myopic focus happens first in the patient's own perspective of their pain. If your back hurts, the first logical thing to do is try and get your back examined and treated. As you go see a physician, a physical therapist, or a chiropractor, more often than not they're going to focus on your back as well. The doctor will probably X-ray your back to see what's happening inside, the physical therapist will give you a sheet of exercises to strengthen your core, and the chiropractor will adjust your back to give you some temporary relief. At best, you may find some relief or receive confirmation about your back pain.

But did any of the practitioners take the time to figure out why your pain is really happening? Did anyone view your body as a whole? Did they put your localized back pain into context to see how it is only part of the whole equation? In Diane's case, the decision to treat the localized pain not only made her knee worse, but as we mentioned before, also caused her to develop nerve symptoms as well as back pain.

It's my belief that only when you see the body in its entire context will you truly understand why the localized pain you're experiencing is actually happening. And only when you consider the context around how your entire body operates will being laser-focused help you treat the area where you're experiencing pain and get the answers you're desperately seeking.

An Artistic Approach to Pain and the Human Body

How can we learn to see the entire picture when it comes to our pain? To answer that I often turn to one of my favorite artists, the impressionist painter George Seurat. He was a leader of the impressionist painting style known as *pointillism*. Pointillism is a technique that uses a series of single, pointed dots painted in different colors on a canvas. When viewing the canvas up close, all you see is a series of colorful dots. But as you step back from the individual points of paint and broaden your perspective, you begin to see that the individual dots create a painting of a beautiful landscape full of color, depth, and imagery spread across the large canvas. Through calculations about how colors work in sequence, each dot works together to create something greater.

One of Seurat's most famous paintings is called *Sunday Afternoon on the Island of La Grande Jatte* (1884). The picture is a composition of Parisian culture, capturing locals spending the day at a park along the banks of the River Seine. The painting is full of natural landscape colors with green, grassy fields, blue sky, and the park's pond where people are boating. In the scene, a little girl holds the hand of her parent while enjoying a walk on a restful Sunday afternoon in the park. One of the most notable things about the work is the facial expression of the little girl taking a stroll in the garden and enjoying the day with her parents. As you get closer and closer to the girl's face, you begin to see how the series of colorful dots work together to make up the beauty of her eyes and reveal the innocence, peace, and joy she's experiencing.

Whenever I see this picture, I can't help but think about how well it captures the way the body is designed. Every joint, every muscle, every part of the body, in and of itself, is an amazing thing that can work independently. But, just like with the George Seurat paintings, if you take a step back, you will see that the entire series of joints, muscles, tendons, ligaments, nerves, fascia, and other structures interactively work together as well. So when we look at pain, we should not look just at the specific point or body part, but we should also take a step back to see the entire landscape of the body.

Here's another way to look at it: for healthcare providers, each specialty represents a different dot within the canvas of the healthcare system. Combining all the vast specialties out there gives us the potential to help a lot of people; however, if there isn't anyone to connect all the dots or coordinate between the different specialists each patient sees, we miss the overarching story. It's as though we're only focusing on the dots that create the girl's eyes and not paying attention to how it all fits into the entire picture.

This is an example of what Diane, and perhaps even you, experienced on a journey through the healthcare system. Every specialist looked at their own dot, but no one saw how it might contribute to the larger picture or the entire flow of the body itself. Conversely, I'm assuming you feel no one has even viewed your body as a whole canvas and realized there is something wrong where a few, small points were not working together correctly, throwing off the entire flow of the picture. Instead, every practitioner focused on the unique points they could treat, and left you feeling like nobody fully understood your body and the bigger picture of your unresolved pain.

Your Movement Story: A Roadmap to the Roots of Your Pain

So how can we see the bigger picture when it comes to your pain? Well, I wrote this book to help you connect the dots.

When it comes to unresolved pain, there is no single body part that can simply be repaired or replaced to fix the problem. Instead, this book will help you understand why the localized pain in your body is a result of the way your entire body functions and moves as a whole. It is a blend between the unique story of who you are and how your pain developed as well as the way your body is designed to be an amazing thing built to function, move, breathe, eat, and live. Not until you understand the balance between your individual story and the design of the body will you be able to see how your pain has come to be what it is. I refer to the process of understanding this balance as your *Movement Story*.

Like pointillism, your Movement Story is the notion that both you and the healthcare system need to see the body as an entire context of interconnected parts that are dependent on one another to work in harmony and achieve the things we're designed to do. To get to the root of your unresolved pain, you need to know your entire Movement Story. Only then will you be able to address the true causes and take the necessary steps toward treatment or intervention to make the unique parts of the whole body work together again.

Simply put:

Your Movement Story

=

your unique pain narrative

+

your body's natural design

This equation includes the notion that there are concrete constructs in the way your body is designed to function and perform; however, that alone is not the full context. If it were, you would be just like a car that could be fixed by changing the parts.

But you're not a car. You're a person with a heart and soul that has journeyed through life. Maybe as a youth you played high-level sports or you were involved in a significant car accident. Maybe you suffered a physically or emotionally traumatic event or you were born with a congenital dysfunction that you have learned to live with. Maybe you've pursued your career dreams, your personal goals, or supported a family.

All of these things make up your unique narrative of who you are, and they make you entirely different from anyone else. The context around the unique narrative of who you are, what you've been through, and what motivates you combines with the nature of your physical body and all of its parts to paint the entire context of your body—physically, emotionally, and spiritually.

Starting now, we'll begin a journey through this book to explore your unresolved pain. Ultimately, my goal is for you to understand your own Movement Story well enough to help you find the answers you've been looking for. I also hope that, through this book, you'll able to redirect your journey with health so you can once again live the life you desire.

KEY POINTS TO REMEMBER:

- In today's healthcare, many health practitioners have their own myopic view about how your body works.

- This myopic view can lead to a confirmation bias that does not identify the entire context of your pain.

- Instead, it is important to know your entire landscape of your pain, known as your Movement Story.

Section 1.2:

Unveiling Your Pain Narrative

What if you were to look beyond the moment you first felt pain? If you looked at the weeks, months, and years leading up to a tweaked back or numbness down your arm, what would you find?

Regardless of whether your pain just started or seems to have been around forever, there is a story or narrative behind it. Everyone's body has a story that began long before their injury occurred. In fact, most injuries are more than a one-time, one-place occurrence. Instead they're often the result of an imbalance you may have unknowingly had for years, or even decades; the manifestation of pain is just the final straw.

What would you find if you were to unravel the complex sequence of events that created your pain narrative? What if retracing that journey from the very beginning could also lead you back to health?

Without exploring the whole narrative, you may live your life in a state of ongoing, or unresolved, pain. You may be puzzled or frustrated when, after a while, the physical therapy, medications, and injections no longer provide even short-term relief. You may eventually give up on treatment. Like most people living with unresolved pain, you may decide to either suffer through the activities that aggravate your pain or simply avoid them altogether.

While avoiding certain things may seem like a feasible solution, it's not a sustainable one. When you opt to avoid painful activities, you risk falling into a fear-avoidance cycle. A fear-avoidance model begins by avoiding movement to prevent pain and leads to disengagement from meaningful activities, which can evolve into other disabilities and depression. Ultimately the fear of pain alone can have a larger impact on your behavior than the pain itself.

Instead of avoiding your pain, knowing your own Movement Story helps you examine it more closely. The process removes the focus from a single pain point and widens the view to include other circumstances that might be contributing. For instance, what appear to be minor, unrelated medical conditions, like asthma, sinus issues, or food sensitivities may actually be tied to your unresolved pain, and misdiagnosed or mistreated pain can evolve into psychological or emotional pain, affecting your ability to work and play.

Taking a more holistic approach may show connections you never considered, and this perspective alone will give you a fighting chance at relieving your unresolved pain for good. When you understand the narrative nature of pain and all the conditions that impact your body, you can objectively see the story behind your unresolved pain and pave a new path toward permanent healing.

How can one so-called "story" have such a big impact? Well, within the context of pain, all body parts are connected. Just because you feel pain in one area, it doesn't necessarily mean that's where it originated. Because the body is built to be symmetrical, any imbalance can lead to injury. So, if you injure your right ankle, the muscles on the left side of your body will work harder to make up for the weakness.

You've probably experienced this phenomenon when carrying groceries. When you carry a heavy bag in one arm, your body will naturally counterbalance the pull by using the muscles on the other side of your body to straighten you out. Being upright, balanced, and symmetrical is your body's primary objective, and it works the same way with injuries.

Unfortunately, some medical professionals tend to overlook this information when treating injuries. While all medical professionals understand the interdependent nature of the body to some extent, ever-changing factors like time, costs, specialization, and insurance coverage encourage most of these professionals to address pain and injury in a singular way.

So, when you tell your primary care physician that your back hurts, they treat your back. If you say you have pain in your shoulder, they order an X-ray of your shoulder. In some cases, the doctor may discover <u>inflammation</u> or damaged tissue, leading them to diagnose the injury and treat you based on what they found. If you're lucky, over time, the swelling goes down and the tissue heals, but the underlying source of the damage goes untreated. In this case the symptoms have been addressed, but the cause is still there.

Of course, this is not an appeal to ignore your current pain— you should absolutely undergo treatment to find relief. But don't let that be your last stop, because this is where knowing your entire Movement Story can make all the difference. By tracking your pain chronologically, you may discover that your first major injury has been the building block for your unresolved pain.

Think about it for a moment: have you ever written down your entire injury history and tried to see whether there might be a correlation between each time you hurt yourself? Or how each incident could have led to the next injury? See if you can draw parallels between your existing pain, your injury history, and any residual effects.

If you did only that, you'd be better informed than many health practitioners, and armed to advocate for your health. While it would be nice if a trained health practitioner mapped your history for you, only you can truly know your body. Understanding your pain narrative will help you take ownership over your care, participate in your appointments, and take the lead in healing all those initial injuries that may have culminated, one by one, in the pain you feel now.

As an example, imagine a person who exercises religiously to avoid weight gain. We'll call him Ben. Perhaps one day Ben pushes a little too hard and injures himself. Not wanting to miss any exercise, he sees a physical therapist who tries to relieve the pain and get Ben moving more effectively. But Ben returns to the same routine only to get hurt again. After digging deeper into why Ben feels the need to exercise so intensely, the therapist learns that his father passed away at just forty-five years old. It turns out Ben's dad was overweight, had high cholesterol, and suffered a heart attack.

Suddenly it makes more sense that Ben, a forty-five-year-old himself, is determined to stay fit in order to avoid meeting the same fate as his father. Perhaps, until the conversation with the physical therapist, Ben hadn't even connected the dots between his father's passing and his own motivations for health. Perhaps this provides an AHA! moment that might have otherwise been missed, and he can finally understand the truth behind his pain, his body, and his goals.

Now, Ben realizes it's not necessarily healthy to be obsessed with exercise either. He realizes it has been taking time away from his own family, which caused additional stress and furthered his unhealthy obsession. Armed with a new perspective, Ben can modify his approach to fitness, learn from the physical therapy, find balance, and feel well enough to enjoy his life again. Consequently, his injury is given the time and space it needs to heal simply because his self-imposed stringency has lessened.

Coming to a realization of this sort is a powerful moment, and it's one I'm lucky to be a part of. I have seen firsthand how understanding your history can give you a renewed sense of ownership, empowerment, and hope. This feeling of ownership is crucial because it creates a connection between the thing we feel control over (in this case, our bodies) and our identities. It enables you to regain your own story, your own pain, and your own life.

Being able to take ownership over your care and participate

more actively in your appointments can help you and your medical practitioners find better solutions together. You can then focus on fixing the things that may be the true culprit, the things that may be the catalyst, for your current pain. Sure, you may you still want to treat your localized pain, but matching it up to your injury history and each residual effect will give you a much better chance at resolving your ongoing pain.

Working in tandem with your health practitioners is akin to paying a financial advisor. It's all well and good to seek a consult, but only you can take full responsibility for the way you save or spend your money—the same is true of your body. You can consult a physician, or even several, but ultimately you have a responsibility to take care of your body—no physician can do that for you. But by finding the right physical therapist, one who really understands your pain, your story, and your goals, you can yield remarkable results. You can come to see a tangible return on your investment, just as you would working with a financial planner.

Without knowing your full pain narrative, you might never uncover what it is that the exercises and treatments are actually trying to heal. You might not even believe that your physical therapist fully understands your pain, because the true cause of your suffering may be buried far beneath the surface of your physical injury. And you wouldn't be wrong. How can anyone fully rehabilitate or heal someone without knowing who the person is as a whole?

Discovering the hidden causes of your pain marks the beginning of a new story: your healing journey. With the entire context of your story, you can see how those little, seemingly trivial injuries created a ripple effect throughout your body's systems. Now you can see that you've been pushing through more than you thought for probably much longer than you thought.

That's why it's essential to have the context that comes from knowing your own Movement Story. Because a single needle in an aching muscle or one injection in your spine cannot fix anything that lies deep within your unresolved pain story. Instead, understanding your history provides you and your physical therapist with a detailed guide for when and where to intervene, enabling you to get out of pain and reach a higher level of performance than you had before. Most importantly, it puts you on a path that could permanently end the pain.

Now that we've established the importance of understanding your own pain narrative, let's get more practical and start applying the method specifically to your body. The next section is designed to be a guide that will help you uncover your own pain narrative. It will require you to take it step by step and break your story into smaller parts. The individual parts we discuss may seem fragmented at first, but my hope is that by bringing it all together in the end, you'll be able to see what your pain narrative is all about. It may take some patience, but don't worry if you don't understand it all by the end of this section; we'll revisit your journey to know your Movement Story throughout the book until it comes together at the end. Let's give it a try.

The Foundation for Your Pain Narrative

To truly understand your bigger pain narrative, you'll need to explore a lot of factors that may seem unrelated at first. We'll need to learn more about your current pain, your injury history, your daily routines and patterns, and even your medical history. All of these play a role in how your body functions, and, as such, all of these things play a role in your pain. To connect all the parts of your pain narrative in a way you can completely understand, we'll break our journey into three parts. First, we'll explore your pain and establish the basic narrative. Then we'll look at your patterns to get an idea of when your pain is better or worse. Finally, we'll look at the history that makes your pain narrative especially unique to you. The rest of this section will go as follows:

1 Uncover Your Pain Narrative

2 Understand Your Pain Patterns

3 Incorporate Your Pain History

1. Uncover Your Pain Narrative

Let's start by uncovering your pain narrative. Without this foundation, you'd be chasing after things, looking for different answers, surfing through "Dr. Web," and grasping at whatever information you can find that may sound like it pertains to you in some way. Instead, this approach is intended to be an easy way for you to apply the idea of your Movement Story specifically to your pain.

In this section, we'll lay down the groundwork to start establishing your pain narrative. The guide allows you to identify where things hurt. At first it may not seem logical to list out a bunch of pain or draw things on paper, but this is your chance to put your story onto a blank canvas. To establish the foundation of your pain story, we're going to draw out your pain and then ask you three basic questions to help filter the different types of pain you may be experiencing. The questions we'll ask include:

A. Where does it hurt?

B. Where else does it hurt?

C. How did you hurt it?

Ready? Let's get started.

Your Body Diagram

First, let's start by giving you a blank canvas on which you can paint your pain narrative. As a visual learner, I abide by the idea that a picture is worth a thousand words. And as a clinician, I use what's called a Body Diagram to help identify specific locations of pain on a patient. I'd encourage you to use the Body Diagram below.

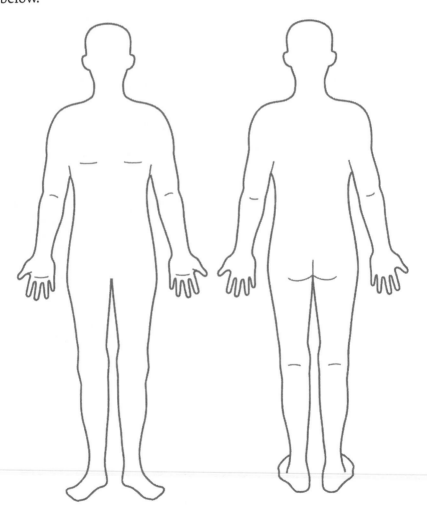

Using the diagram, I simply want you to draw your pain or the symptoms you are currently experiencing. Feel free to be as expressive and detailed as you'd like. It might also help to be clear about the symptoms that are sharp and localized by drawing a distinct X on the spot where you can pinpoint shoulder or knee pain, for example.

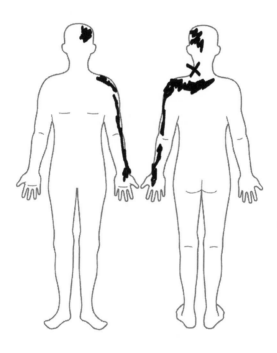

Or perhaps you have a long history of tingling, numbness, or burning sensations down your leg or arm. In that case, feel free to draw squiggly lines or shade in pencil marks along the arm or leg to depict the nerve-related symptoms you're feeling from your spine down to your fingertips or toes.

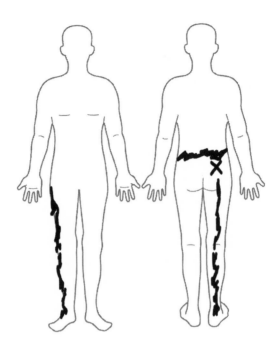

Perhaps you have more diffuse pain that spans across your entire mid and low back. Here, you may want to scribble in or circle broadly where your pain is since it's not a distinct pain, like shoulder pain you can pinpoint, but a broader, more diffuse pain. This is the kind that makes doctors scratch their heads a bit and think it must be chronic, non-specific, or insidious back pain, or even possibly the dreaded fibromyalgia.

Either way, it's important you take this time to be honest about it because this is *your* pain and no one else's. No one else can describe the symptoms as well as you can. So, make sure when you finish drawing, the diagram effectively symbolizes the pain or the symptoms you're experiencing. Once you feel confident about identifying your pain, we can ask our clarifying questions.

A. Where does it hurt? Primary Pain Complaints

Now that you've drawn out your pain, I also want you to write about it using words and phrases that best describe it. I'd encourage you to take time to write a list of all the pains and symptoms you're experiencing. But more than just listing them, I also want you to describe what each symptom feels like. For example:

INJURY: Sciatica down my right leg.

DESCRIPTION: It feels numb and sometimes burns all the way down to my toes.

Now, you try:

INJURY:

DESCRIPTION:

INJURY:

DESCRIPTION:

This description of what we'll call your *primary pain complaints* helps us establish the main areas that are currently causing the most discomfort or dissonance in your body. Using the previous example of artist George Seurat's pointillism, this is maybe just one or two colorful points, but it does not make up the whole canvas. In your case, it may or may not be the reason you're experiencing pain. But being aware of it creates a focal point we can target to measure your progress. If you have multiple areas of pain, try to prioritize the one that seems to be the most problematic *right now*. In the next section, we can add any other symptoms you have.

B. Where else does it hurt?
Secondary Pain Complaints

Once you've described your persistent, nagging pains in detail, we'll continue with another exercise. This time, I want you to write down any other pains you are currently experiencing or have recently experienced, but that are not as prominent or bothersome as your primary pain complaint. These symptoms, which we'll call *secondary pain complaints*, include the pains you've been able to live with or don't feel as problematic or aggravating as the pains you listed first.

These secondary symptoms may seem small or insignificant to you, but more often than not, there is a surprising correlation between primary and secondary pain complaints. You may even want to draw your secondary pain complaints on your body diagram in another color. If you do, make sure you clearly depict it as separate from your primary pain complaints so you know the difference when you refer back to it. Then, just as before, take time to write down where the secondary pain complaints hurt and describe how they feel. For example:

INJURY: ___Left shoulder pain._____

DESCRIPTION: ___Localized and sharp when I raise my arm.___
_____

Now, it's your turn:

INJURY: _____

DESCRIPTION: _____
_____

INJURY: _____

DESCRIPTION: _____
_____

Remember to do this once for *every* secondary pain complaint you have.

C. How did you hurt it? Mechanism of Injury

After you've listed all of your pain complaints, there is one more step to establishing the foundation for your pain narrative. Now you have to ask yourself, "How did I hurt it?"

Again, it's important to take your time to describe how you think your pain came to be. In clinical terminology we call this catalyst the *Mechanism of Injury*, and we use it to define whether there is a specific cause or reason for your pain or injury. Remember to write down the mechanism of injury for both your primary and secondary pain complaints. Then, once you've written them down, I'd also like you to categorize your pain in one of three ways, as either traumatic, repetitive, or insidious. What's the difference?

A traumatic injury can be defined as one that takes place during an event that was more abrupt in nature or was caused by an unexpected force. This sort of injury would include a car accident or a contact-sports injury, like being tackled in football or tripped in soccer. Some self-induced injuries fall into this category, too, like throwing out your back by lifting a heavy box or rolling your ankle by stepping off a curb.

Repetitive or prolonged injuries, on the other hand, are those that happen as a result of doing something repeatedly over a sustained amount of time. This could be something like getting an elbow injury by playing too much tennis or by hammering all day long to install a new deck. This category could also include postural injuries. With much of Western society working at desks all day, it could include the tightness or pain you feel in your back or neck when you sit too long. Or, even with the use of modern standing desks, the dull, achy, and diffuse pain you feel in your neck or back could be classified as a repetitive injury.

Finally, insidious injuries are basically any injuries that do not fall into the other two categories, traumatic or repetitive. These are the injuries for which you cannot determine the precise moment they took place and you have no idea where they came from. As we begin this journey together, it's possible that there will be more injuries classified as insidious-onset injuries than anything else because you might not fully understand where your pain came from. These types of pain are the ones you noticed when you woke up one day and they had magically appeared, seemingly without rhyme or reason. But because of their ambiguity, they may be a symptom of an issue that's not muscular or orthopedic in nature, and therefore insidious onset injuries need to be explored more carefully. From time to time, some more serious medical diagnoses can manifest as physical pain that you may simply misunderstand as a muscular strain.

If you're unsure whether your pain might be medically related, I'd recommend contacting your physician to have any underlying conditions ruled out; however, assuming your pain is muscular or orthopedic in nature, you'll want to take time to write down how you think it came to be. For example:

INJURY: Low back spasm

CATEGORY: Traumatic

MECHANISM: Lifting a box

Now, it's your turn.

INJURY: _____

CATEGORY: _____

MECHANISM: _____

INJURY: _____

CATEGORY: _____

MECHANISM: _____

Remember to do this exercise for both primary *and* secondary complaints.

As you log your injuries, you may notice that traumatic injuries are easier to process because there is usually a clear cause or reason why the pain began. Repetitive or prolonged injuries sometimes can be harder to identify. Although there may be a cause you can point to, repetitive injuries are usually those that make you wonder, "If I've been able to do this exercise without a problem before, why would it be painful now?" Like repetitive injuries, insidious-onset injures can also be difficult to determine.

It can range from a medical issue (which I hope is not the case) to pain caused by any reason you can't pinpoint.

In either case, my hope is that through this book, we'll be able to get to the bottom of those nebulous injuries so they make more sense to you. In the end, the more sense those injuries make, the more likely you'll be able to move forward and get better.

Summarizing the Foundation of Your Pain Narrative

Now that you've taken the time to draw out your pain, write it down, establish what your primary and secondary pain complaints are, and try to determine where they came from, you should be able to step back and see, more holistically, everything that you've uncovered.

When I examine my patients for the first time and we go through all the exercises you've just completed, it helps lay a baseline, or foundation, for the types of pain the patient is experiencing. At this point I likely still have little knowledge about the extent of or the causes behind the pain, but this process helps set the stage so that, as we explore their story further, we can build upon it. Having this foundation is crucial to developing the rest of your pain narrative, so, if you rushed through this section, I'd encourage you to go back and take your time fully describing and detailing the pain you're experiencing and how you think it may have begun.

NOTES

2. Understand Your Pain Patterns

Now that we have a basic understanding of your pain, what it feels like, and where it came from, we can move on to creating more clarity around how your pain behaves. In clinical terms we call this the *nature of your pain*. By now you know that not all pain is the same; therefore, it's important to be able to clearly define the type of pain you are experiencing. The types are not only determined by the symptoms you feel—whether they are sharp, diffuse, burning, achy, etc.—but also by when the pain occurs.

Because much of the pain you're experiencing is more clearly defined by when it happens in addition to what you feel, it leads us to ask our next clarifying question: When does it hurt? In our clinical examination, we use two main categories to help describe the nature of your pain. They include:

- Aggravating and Easing Factors
- Your 24-Hour Pain Pattern

Let's explore what these categories mean in terms of your pain.

Aggravating Factors

Focusing on your primary pain complaints, let's go through an exercise to help determine what makes your pain better or worse. It's simple: just write down two or three things that make your pain worse, and how long it takes to worsen.

Hopefully you won't have to search for these things. They should be the things you do while going about your daily life, playing a specific sport, or performing a certain activity that causes you pain. For example, oftentimes people experiencing low-back pain will have more pain if they sit for too long, and bending forwards may make their pain worse.

Similarly, if your pain worsens over time or during a specific activity, I'd like you to write down the activity as well as the time it takes for your pain to occur. Using the sitting example, you would write down how long you can sit before your low back starts to hurt, which is maybe something like 15 to 20 minutes.

In some cases, the time parameter might need to be determined more objectively. With runners, for example, it may not necessarily be a certain amount of time that passes, but rather the number of laps around the track or a certain incline on a treadmill. Or with high-intensity interval trainers, it may be a specific type of squat using a specific amount of weight or the number of repetitions that causes pain. With golfers, it may be the number of holes or swings.

Either way, I want you to be able to write down a tangible time, sport, or activity that lets you quantify, as precisely as possible, when your pain takes place. It may not be clearly cut or defined, but do your best to create as much clarity as possible. For example:

INJURY: Low-back spasm

AGGRAVATING ACTIVITY: Sitting

TIMEFRAME: 20 minutes

Or

INJURY: Knee pain

AGGRAVATING ACTIVITY: Playing golf

TIMEFRAME: 12th hole

Now, once again, it's your turn:

INJURY:

AGGRAVATING ACTIVITY:

TIMEFRAME:

INJURY:

AGGRAVATING ACTIVITY:

TIMEFRAME:

Easing Factors

Just as knowing what makes your pain worse helps you understand your pain, so does knowing what makes it feel better. So, for this exercise, I want you to write down two or three things that either get rid of your pain or at least decrease it enough to be bearable.

No doubt there are times that your pain feels relentless; sometimes it hurts constantly and never goes away. You might often feel consumed by your pain, but take time to really think about moments when your pain is more tolerable compared to other times when it's completely horrible. Even with more chronic or unresolved pain, there are typically times when the pain ebbs and flows or feels calmer than usual.

For example, with the case of low-back pain, walking for short periods or laying down to rest can often ease that pain. Although that's not a long-term solution, it does establish that your pain can be calmed to some extent. Any relief, no matter how brief, should be recognized and noted as information about the nature of your pain. I'd encourage you to take time to write down any easing factors. Additionally, if you have a sense for the duration or another measure that defines how long it takes for your pain to ease, write that down as well. For example:

INJURY: Low-back pain

EASING ACTIVITY: Short walks

TIMEFRAME: 15 minutes

Or

INJURY: Neck pain

EASING ACTIVITY: Laying down

TIMEFRAME: 30 minutes

Now, it's your turn:

INJURY:

EASING ACTIVITY:

TIMEFRAME:

INJURY:

EASING ACTIVITY:

TIMEFRAME:

It may seem obvious that defining your aggravating and easing factors can help you determine specific activities that make your pain better or worse. More importantly, this helps us look at those activities to figure out what specifically makes it better or worse so we can then ask, "How can we make your body work so you can do that activity without getting hurt?"

In the back pain example, if sitting causes pain, we probably want to look at your workstation to create an ergonomic space that lessens the stress on your body. We may also determine that your physical body, due to some type of tightness or weakness, simply does not have the capacity to sit for eight or more hours every day.

Similarly, if golfing hurts after twelve holes, we need to look at your swing technique, as it may cause your body to fatigue and create extraneous forces that lead to back or neck pain, and we also need to consider your flexibility and strength to handle the swing itself. In addition to improving your swing, improving both your technique and your physical fitness can help you feel less pain as well.

24-Hour Pattern

Another way to look at the nature of your pain is not based on the activities that may provoke or decrease it, but rather on looking more broadly at your entire day. How does your pain behave throughout the day, from morning to evening, or at nighttime while you're sleeping? As it relates to your pain, we call this your 24-hour pattern.

This 24-hour pattern examines what your pain looks and feels like around the clock, twenty-four hours a day, seven days a week. Again, there may be times when your pain feels incessant, like it constantly hurts and never subsides. But in many cases of unresolved pain, there is an underlying pattern for when your pain occurs. Even though it may feel like your pain is noticeable all the time, we can uncover times it's more or less intense by asking the right questions.

Start by thinking about a normal day in your life. Maybe you wake up, do your morning routine, go to work, and do all the things you typically do there. Perhaps you work out after a long day at work, come home, settle down, and go to sleep for the night. Now think about the trends or patterns that happen during your routine. Especially if your pain has been present for a while and you've gotten so used to it that you don't notice when it gets worse or better, take time to ask yourself these clarifying questions:

- How does my pain feel when I first wake up in the morning? Is it really sharp and intense? Or is it dull and achy? Is it really bad or not that bad?

- How does my pain feel as I wake up and get moving? If I have pain when I wake up, does it take a long time for it to loosen up and shake off? Or does it decrease quickly as I get out of bed?

- How does my pain feel as the day goes on? Around early afternoon, on a typical day, how does my pain behave? Is it painful all morning and gets worse as the day goes on? Or is my pain not that bad in the morning, but by mid- to late afternoon I find it worsening? By the time I come home, am I in excruciating pain?

- When I am home in the evening, is my pain bearable, depending on what activities I performed that day? Or is it so intense that, no matter what, I am just begging to crawl into bed and call it a night?

- What about when I am sleeping? Am I able to sleep through the night without a problem or does my pain wake me up? If I wake up, is it easy to fall back to sleep or does my pain keep me up all night?

Thinking through these questions should help you clarify when exactly your pain occurs instead of thinking it's there all the time. Establishing your 24-hour pattern provides information about the severity of your pain and answering these questions can help us understand what factors may worsen your pain. The timing will often help us determine whether it's tied to your nerves or whether there are specific activities that provoke it. So, let's look at what the timing of your pain during a 24-hour cycle means, starting with the morning.

Morning

People who experience sharper pain first thing in the morning are typically dealing with issues of acute inflammation. Think of a time you maybe sprained your ankle or wrist and you saw a pocket of fluid buildup. That fluid is a result of inflammation.

Typically, inflammation increases when you rest and sleep. So, when you wake up in the morning, the inflammation that has built up during your sleep is greater and it provokes your pain in a very sharp and distinct way, making it hard to even get out of bed. On the other hand, pain that's duller and more achy is not as severe and indicates a more chronic, but less acute, inflamed state.

Afternoon and Evening

Pain that worsens as the day goes on, rather than first thing in the morning, can be interesting for its own reasons. Some patients will come in and say, "At 2 P.M. I know the pain in my back or neck is coming. It happens so regularly, that I plan my day around it and get all of my chores done early, so when the pain strikes at 2 P.M., I can call it a day." And while there may not be a clear time when your pain begins, you might find that your pain worsens during your daily routine. Especially if your pain is not as bad in the morning, your afternoon pain indicates that your body is fatiguing and losing its stamina to perform your everyday activities.

If you're thinking, "Does that mean I'm not strong enough to make it through the day?" in most cases, the answer is no. You're strong enough to make it through the day, but your pain is a sign of fatigue. It's not unlike a runner who's only conditioned to run five miles, but keeps running twenty miles to train for a marathon. If you keep exhausting yourself by running more than you're used to, a lack of muscle endurance and conditioning will more than likely lead to pain.

Sleeping

What's happening when you're unable to sleep through the night, or when your pain wakes you up from an otherwise sound sleep? Well, with respect to medical safety, pain that occurs while you sleep can be an indicator of more sinister or pathologic pain patterns, though the pain is usually paired with other notable symptoms like extreme weight loss, extreme weight gain, or other neurological symptoms such as, but not limited to, numbness, tingling, burning, or tremors. If you're experiencing any of those symptoms, you should contact your physician to rule out other pathologic problems.

If your pain isn't accompanied by other notable symptoms, nighttime pain can be a result of your sleep position. For example, lying on your stomach can increase back pain because it puts too much pressure on your back. Lying on your side can also cause hip or shoulder pain. In this case, the pressure on either side touching the mattress or your side facing upward can be aggravated by the position. Sometimes just using pillows or other forms of support can help take pressure off the joints.

Other times, the pain you get at night is an accumulation from the activities you did the day before. It may not have hurt much during the day or as you did your activities, but it may worsen as your body settles at rest. As with afternoon and evening pain, this kind of pain indicates that your body is fatiguing earlier than expected. Perhaps you were doing a repetitive or prolonged activity that your body didn't have the stamina to handle. That kind of injury can start an inflammatory cycle and cause pain at night.

As you think about your 24-hour pattern, ask yourself how your pain feels throughout your day. Know that each of these factors will give us clues about what's causing your pain, and take your time writing down how your pain behaves during the following times of day:

MORNING:

_____

_____

AFTERNOON / EVENING:

_____

_____

SLEEPING:

_____

_____

As we continue to explore your pain narrative, you'll put all of this together along with the other factors you're writing down. Hopefully, by the end, you'll have more clarity about your pain instead of just inferring what a scan says about you.

Summarizing Your Pain Patterns

At this point, you should already know much more about your pain narrative. You've established the foundation by drawing your pain, describing it, and determining how it began, whether through traumatic, repetitive, or insidious reasons, and you've explored the nature of your pain by describing what makes it worse, what makes it better, and how it behaves through a 24-hour pattern. While, in some cases, your pain may not be so simple to describe, I'd encourage you to note as much as you can. As we continue, these exercises will reveal more clarity around your pain narrative and help you find relief.

NOTES

_____

_____

_____

_____

_____

_____

_____

3. Incorporate Your Pain History

One of the most important things about your pain is that it is *yours*. While it's true that everyone may suffer from pain at some point, almost no one suffers in the same way or for the same reasons. Simply put: everyone sits, everyone stands, and everyone lifts things; pain happens to essentially everyone. So, what makes your pain unique? Why do you have unresolved pain when a friend or colleague who once had similar pain got better?

In short, your pain is unique because you are unique. And because no two life experiences are the same, part of understanding your pain story involves getting more detailed. It's important to determine the things that are unique about you, including who you are, what you've done, what you do now, and what motivates you, as your motivations can often become an unconscious driver behind the reasons you're experiencing unresolved pain.

As the last step in learning your pain story, we'll take a closer look at three factors in this section. They include:

- Your medical history;
- Your activity history; and
- Your motivating factors.

Let's start with your medical history.

Medical History

I don't think anyone enjoys filling out long hospital forms about their medical history. But there's a reason health practitioners ask you if you have previous or existing medical conditions. It informs health practitioners about any precautions they should take, advises against treatments that could make you worse, and sends warning signs for different ailments you may be experiencing. A skilled health practitioner should have the capacity to understand a medical or injury history and put it into context around the issue you're presenting with when they see you. As with the other exercises in this book, it's equally important to take your time describing your medical history to the best of your ability.

When it comes to your pain narrative, listing your medical history goes beyond indicating whether you have high cholesterol or occasional vertigo. Instead, it can be broken down into four main categories, including:

- Injury history;
- Surgical history;
- Medical conditions; and
- Structural abnormalities.

Injury History

Let's start with your previous injuries. The reason you should keep a list of your injuries is simple: oftentimes there is a correlation between injuries that seem unrelated. So, even if all your past injuries were in your lower body and your current pain is localized to your upper body, there may be a clear correlation between the number of ankle sprains you've experienced and your more recent neck pain.

It's important to try and remember as much as you can for this exercise, so for the next exercise, take your time to list any injuries you've had, in chronological order, either by the year it happened or the age you were at the time. Remember to specify which side of the body as well. For example:

INJURY: Sprained right ankle _____

WHEN: Eight years old _____

Or

INJURY: Left ACL tear _____

WHEN: 2005 _____

Now start your list:

INJURY: _____

WHEN: _____

INJURY: _____

WHEN: _____

INJURY: _____

WHEN: _____

INJURY: _____

WHEN: _____

Surgical History

Your surgical history also tells us a lot about how your body works. Obviously there are varying levels of severity, between spraining an ankle and having surgery that required plates and screws, but there is usually a significant reason why a physician decides to perform surgery. From a functional perspective, anytime an incision is made, more inflammation is caused, both by the trauma of the injury and by the surgery itself. The more inflammation that occurs and the larger or deeper the incision, the more likely scar tissue is to form—and scar tissue, in and of itself, can be a driver in your pain and dysfunction.

To help identify any possible connections, take time to write down your surgical history. Just like you did with your previous injuries, do your best to list everything you can in chronological order by the year or the age you were when it took place. The list should include surgeries that are not just orthopedic in nature, such as back surgery or rotator cuff repairs, but also any other surgeries you had for medical or elective reasons.

Common surgeries that should be listed might include: abdominal surgeries, chest surgeries—whether for respiratory conditions or breast reconstruction—sinus surgeries and other orofacial procedures, hernia repair, or any surgeries you may have forgotten about. Again, remember to specify the side of the body, whenever applicable. For example:

SURGERY: Back surgery, L4-S1

WHEN: 2009

Now write your list:

SURGERY:

WHEN:

SURGERY:

WHEN:

SURGERY:

WHEN:

SURGERY:

WHEN:

Medical Conditions

While I'm not a physician, I know that understanding your medical history is vital to treating unresolved pain. Not only can your internal medical history indicate other reasons you might be experiencing physical pain, but it might also have something to do with why you're experiencing orthopedic pain. Too many times we separate internal medicine diagnoses from orthopedic diagnoses, when we should always consider the possibility of a correlation or a relationship between them. As such, this is a good time to list any major medical conditions you have along with the time they began. For example:

CONDITION: Diabetes

WHEN: 2013

Once again, it's your turn:

CONDITION: _____

WHEN: _____

CONDITION: _____

WHEN: _____

CONDITION: _____

WHEN: _____

CONDITION: _____

WHEN: _____

Below are some of the most common medical pathologies that can correlate to unresolved musculoskeletal pain:

Issues related to your internal organs, such as reflux and food or mold sensitivities. Inflamed internal organs, for example, may cause more inflammation and pain in other areas of your body, like your mid-back. Sometimes inflammation chemicals can travel from your spine into your arms, legs, hands or feet, causing a burning pain. These feelings are known as <u>antegrade impulses</u>, and just as inflammatory chemicals travel away from your spine, your nerve also has the capacity to send inflammatory mediators the opposite direction. That means if your internal organs are inflamed, they can send chemical mediators back up the thoracic nerves and into the thoracic spine, causing an inflammatory state in your back.

Respiratory issues like asthma can contribute to neck and shoulder pain as well as recurring tension headaches. What happens is this: your *diaphragm*, the dome-shaped, muscular tissue that separates your chest from your abdominal cavity, is the principal muscle of respiration. Because of its makeup and location, the strength of your <u>diaphragm</u> can also influence your core stability. So, if your breathing becomes limited by your diaphragm, your body resorts to breathing primarily from your upper chest and ribs.

In turn, this action causes you to use your upper chest and neck muscles to breathe—something you do subconsciously nearly every second—instead of using your diaphragm. This coping strategy is called <u>apical breathing</u>, and if it becomes your normal breathing pattern, accessory breathing requires your neck and shoulders to be the source of your breathing capacity. But increasing the workload of these muscles eventually exhausts them more readily, reducing their bandwidth and leading to lingering tension and possible neck pain.

Structural Abnormalities

While you probably haven't been asked to list your structural abnormalities on standard medical history forms, just like medical conditions, they can also influence how efficiently your body moves and functions. Any sense of abnormality or offset in how you're structured can be a foundation for why your pain continues to occur.

Remember Diane? Her leg-length discrepancy caused a persisting knee and nerve pain someone with relatively equal length legs would be less prone to. The most common structural variances tend to be leg lengths and <u>scoliosis</u>, which is a structural twist in the spine, though usually we can see these kinds of structural variances in the way someone walks. Much like a strange use of color in a Seurat painting, structural variances can stand out quite obviously, and even the smallest point of distortion can affect the entire picture.

Sometimes it starts early in our lives, as a pigeon-toed or bow-legged child. Maybe a patient wore corrective shoes or braces on their hips when they were young and never related that history to their current pain complaints. Even if you only had a structural dysfunction as a baby, listing it could show how it became the first building block in your pain story. It may not be the sole reason you're in pain, but it may be the first focal point where your body found a reason to adapt so it could keep moving, running, and getting through the day.

Whether your foot was turned inward so sharply you had to wear a corrective shoe, or you walked with your feet and knees turned outward, you simply learned to live with these things and the fact that some joints pointed the wrong direction may have caused the rest of your leg, your back, and even your arms to work differently. Just like Diane, whose outward-pointing foot resulted in knee pain, you have to consider all of the contributing factors. For this exercise, take the time to list any structural abnormalities and the time you became aware of them, whether treated or untreated. For example:

ABNORMALITY: Leg-length discrepancy

WHEN: Eight years old

Now list yours:

ABNORMALITY: _____

WHEN: _____

ABNORMALITY: _____

WHEN: _____

ABNORMALITY: _____

WHEN: _____

ABNORMALITY: _____

WHEN: _____

Structural asymmetries, usually dependent upon genetics or just plain luck, are imbalances in the body that force changes in length and stability on the surrounding muscles, creating further imbalances that cause pain. Below is a list of common structural abnormalities that correlate to unresolved pain:

While a true discrepancy in structural leg length is uncommon, physical therapists and chiropractors will sometimes say you have a functional leg-length discrepancy. **Functional leg-length discrepancies** are created by a progressive muscle imbalance that pulls your muscles and joints in different directions, so it only appears you have one leg longer than the other. You might find relief by yanking on the leg, but you'll still need to focus on treating the origin of the muscle imbalances to really correct it.

The hips can also suffer from a structural asymmetry, and there are two types of imbalances: anteversion or retroversion. **Hip Anteversion** is often described by the term knock-kneed, and it basically refers to people who walk with their knees turned inward, toward one another. Along with inward-turned knees, people with hip anteversion may also have toes that point inward too. More specifically, hip anteversion means the hip (or hips) sits in its socket at an angle that's turned inward 15 to 20 degrees more than it would be normally.

Because of the joint structure, you may not see the 20-degree inward turn at the hip as clearly as you would see the inward turn at the knees and feet. Still, if left untreated, hip anteversion can place added stress on the leg, change the muscle balance of the hip, and cause pain anywhere from the hip to the pelvis, low back, mid back, and even the neck. This pain can present itself unevenly as well, appearing more on the inside of the anteverted leg and causing medial knee pain, ACL tears, or plantar fasciitis.

In contrast, **hip retroversion** refers to people who have hips that turn outward from their sockets, as though they're seated on a saddle. Like anteverted hips, retroverted hips can also place unnecessary force on the legs; however, <u>retroversion</u> usually appears more commonly on the back and the side of the hip as opposed to the inner leg. In this case the 15- to 20-degree outward turn causes a greater pull on the outside or back of the leg. Thus, people with retroversion imbalances are more likely to experience deep buttock pain like piriformis syndrome or lateral knee pain like IT Band syndrome.

It goes without saying that hip anteversion or retroversion can place a tremendous amount of stress on the hips as well as on the rest of the body. And if one hip is significantly anteverted or retroverted compared to the other, the asymmetry creates a disproportionate amount of stress on one side of the body rather than evenly. Conversely, it can also place asymmetrical stress on the opposite side of the upper body as it tries to coordinate with the imbalance in the hip.

You can test for retroversion or anteversion by simply examining how you sit. Someone with retroverted hips usually sits with one or both legs splayed out from their body, like a frog, so the retroverted leg(s) can open up. Meanwhile, someone with anteverted hips will typically sit with their knees turned inward and their heels turned out underneath them, making a sort of W shape. They might be able to sit on their knees from kneeling position, leaving the ankle and shin turned outward, away from their body.

In either instance, turning your feet in one direction or the other requires a substantial rotation of the hip socket and thigh bone, and it can be difficult, if not impossible, to fully correct a structural imbalance of this type. When accurately diagnosed, however, physical therapists can provide exercises and hands-on techniques to improve the stress caused by both anteversion and retroversion. Fortunately, this is true for most of the predisposing factors we've explored.

Knowing that it can be difficult to uncover the relationship between these predisposing conditions and your existing pain makes it even more important to consider them. While there are many people who live with an asymmetry or imbalance that causes added stress on the body, it's important to know that our bodies can withstand much of it by itself. It's usually only when the asymmetries are tested further in sports or prolonged positions that they can lower our physical threshold. That's why the goal of physical therapy is to reduce asymmetrical stresses by promoting better muscle control, length, and flexibility, creating a higher capacity for withstanding forces and minimizing injuries. So, let's keep working toward that.

Summarizing Your Medical History

Now that you've organized your medical history into four categories (previous injuries, previous surgeries, previous medical conditions, and previous structural abnormalities), you should have a pretty robust list of all the things your body has experienced. While it may be intimidating or discouraging to see a laundry list of issues, it's important to know that each of these can be vital to explaining your unresolved pain. And having this information, combined with the remaining pieces, will hopefully help you find relief.

NOTES

_____

_____

_____

_____

_____

_____

_____

Activity History

Just like your medical history is unique to you, the sports or activities you performed throughout your life may have a direct influence on why your pain is occurring. As youth sports are becoming increasingly competitive, they're often overdone. Surely you can imagine a ten-year-old boy who plays as the star pitcher on his baseball team year-round, aiming to be the next Nolan Ryan, Goose Gossage, or Clayton Kershaw, only to throw out his arm before he gets to high school.

This is especially risky during the developmental years of adolescence, as we're going through puberty, growth spurts, and our muscles, joints, and ligaments are still morphing, growing, and altering to maturation toward adulthood. At the same time, we find ourselves competing at a high level, practicing endless hours, throwing balls, sprinting down fields or tracks, hitting the same tennis ball or volleyball countless times. This strain also pertains to performing arts, like ballerinas who turn out their feet to plié and then go on to pointe, or cheerleaders who do the splits while being thrown into the air for a double flip.

Of course, it's hard to draw a line on pursuing your dreams or mastering a sport or art when the achievement of success can outweigh some of the costs. And sometimes the costs are felt during the time you train, whether in the form of a ligament tear, a fracture, a concussion, or something less traumatic, like repetitive ankle sprains, recurring shin splints, or chronic back spasms. Fortunately, in most cases, our adolescent bodies have the capacity to heal faster than they do as adults.

Yet rarely do we think that the tenth time we sprain our ankle will have a lasting effect on how the rest of our body works for the rest of our lives, or that the spine fracture we got from landing on our back in a bad fall during gymnastics or while being tripped in soccer could have something to do with why we're now experiencing unresolved pain. Over time, any repetition in practicing a sport can alter your body's joints, ligaments, and bone structure.

Perhaps a soccer player who predominantly kicks with his right foot will see his left shin begin to bow outward over time. This is due to the excessive force he put on his left leg to stand firmly enough to allow his right leg to kick the ball. Or in my case, I played competitive tennis for years, and I had a really good serve that could spin the ball to draw people off the side of the court. Then, I simply learned to deal with the sharp pain I sometimes felt in my shoulder. But now, in my mid-forties, I find that my left shoulder is stiffer than my right, I have a harder time reaching behind my back on that side, and I get occasional pain in my left arm.

Moreover, as athletes compete at much higher levels or play much longer, the repetition is increasingly a factor in how their bodies begin to change shape. These are the people we tend to see with ongoing shoulder pain or leg pain later in life, all because of the repercussions from playing sports or pursuing an activity for years. It's simply part of the lives we live; however, only by being mindful of these impacts will you be able to clearly assess whether those years of competition contribute to the pain you have now.

As with the previous histories you listed, take time to write down any high-level sports, performances, or activities you participated in over the years, as well as how long you stayed with them. For example:

ACTIVITY: Soccer

DURATION: 12 years

Now write yours:

ACTIVITY:

DURATION:

ACTIVITY:

DURATION:

ACTIVITY:

DURATION:

Motivating Factors

In the same way your pain stems from who you are physically, it also stems from who you are emotionally and spiritually. Our next exercise in defining your pain story deals with the core of who you are; not necessarily who you are physically, but who you are in your soul. Because, again, we're not made up of interchangeable car parts or Lego pieces we can swap out; who you are determines your unique pain story. This not only relates to the intrinsic interaction of joints, ligaments, muscles, tendons, nerves, and fascia that work together and allow us to move; it also relates to the intrinsic nature of who we are in our hearts and souls.

It may sound corny, but I have been amazed by the number of patients who come into my clinic with ongoing knee pain, back pain, or nerve symptoms because they do a high-intensity workout six days a week. Exercises like squats, burpees, lunges, kettlebells, and sprinting on high-incline treadmills are all designed to help you reach your target heart rate and some classes put you on a score on the board to rank who is the strongest. But they can lead high-achieving personality types to push themselves harder and harder to be number one.

What these patients don't realize is that their physical bodies cannot always withstand that amount of exertion. Just like a paperclip, if you keep bending it back and forth, something will eventually wear out or break. It may sound obvious, but many patients will deny their overuse when I tell them they're pushing way too hard in their classes or workouts.

As I dive deeper into why they're so resistant, it becomes obvious that the patient has an internal factor that drives them to work out feverishly. It may be related to body image issues, losing a parent early due to cardiac reasons, or experiencing abuse as a child that made them feel they would never be good enough. While I'm not a counselor, I know these seeds of belief, value, and motivation can become anchors in what drive people physically and cause them pain. Although this is not a book on the psychology of pain, it's important to raise the issue of motivating factors as context for who you are and how they contribute to your pain narrative.

Even the world's best athletes can struggle with their inner identity that fuels them to perform. Sometimes that ultra-competitive spirit is based on something unhealthy. For instance, tennis star Andre Agassi has written about finding purpose in playing without the weight of his over-abusive father that initially defined him into a life of fame and drugs.[1] Former NBA star Landry Fields shares how his success on the court became an idol to him. Not until his injuries stopped him from playing basketball did he realize that winning on the court was being more valued than what should have been truly important to him: his own Christian faith in God.[2]

Take time to reflect and truly think about who you are, what motivates you, and what fears you have. Ask yourself what deep-seated beliefs you have about yourself that may fuel your goals and ambitions. Ask yourself, like Andre Agassi and Landry Fields did, whether you are healthy or worthy or if you may be an idol, an addiction, or something truly not purposeful. If possible, try to also identify where those beliefs come from. For example:

MOTIVATION: "I have to win!" mentality

SOURCE: Body image issues

Once again, it's your turn to describe your story:

MOTIVATION: _____

SOURCE: _____

MOTIVATION: _____

SOURCE: _____

MOTIVATION: _____

SOURCE: _____

KEY POINTS TO REMEMBER:

- **Global, not just local:** Rather than just rely on a single test or diagnosis to describe your pain, it is important to understand your pain narrative that provides a fuller context of how your pain is behaving.

- **Look back:** Trace back how your symptoms began and how they behave, and get to know your past pain history.

- **It's in your head:** Recognize that your own mindset and what motivates you to move can be, at times, the primary driver of your pain.

Section 1.3:

The Basics of Why Pain Occurs

Now that you've taken the time to describe your unresolved pain, my hope is that you're able to differentiate between the types, locations, and potential causes rather than seeing your pain as an obscure, overarching thing. The next step is to try and make sense of everything you described in the previous section, including:

- What hurts?
- Where does it hurt?
- How did you hurt it?
- When does it hurt? and
- Who are you?

That means that, following the basic themes of storytelling, we've asked: who, what, where, when, and how. The only question we haven't asked yet is "*Why?* Why does it hurt?"

This is the million-dollar question. Because, as you already know, understanding why you have unresolved pain is not as easy as simply looking at a scan and having surgery; it is much more complex than that. In this section, we're going to focus on helping you understand why pain occurs. Using your descriptions of who, what, where, when, and how, we'll be able to zero in on why you're experiencing unresolved pain. Let's get started.

Your Movement Story Graph: Visualizing the Timeline of Your Unresolved Pains

The unfortunate truth is that many of us have very little understanding of how the body works; what it's made of, how everything inside is connected, and what happens as it functions. To help you better understand it, we're going to take this time to talk in depth about what happens in your body whenever you feel pain. At times, what you read may get technical, so hang in there, and remember you can always refer to the glossary at the end of the book for clarification. And don't skip ahead, because knowing precisely what's going on your body is vital to grasping the extent of any issue you might have.

It's important because your body is always working in some way, no matter what you do every day. Though much of it is subconscious, your body is constantly moving. Even if you're not an athlete, daily tasks like brushing your teeth, washing the dishes, and even checking your phone require muscle movement. They may be minute movements, but they all play a role in how the rest of your body moves. Your normal, daily activities set the benchmark for your <u>Movement Story Graph (MSG)</u>.

What exactly is your Movement Story Graph? Essentially your Movement Story Graph is a visual representation that shows your body's everyday physical abilities and its capacity to handle differing loads and stresses.[3,4]

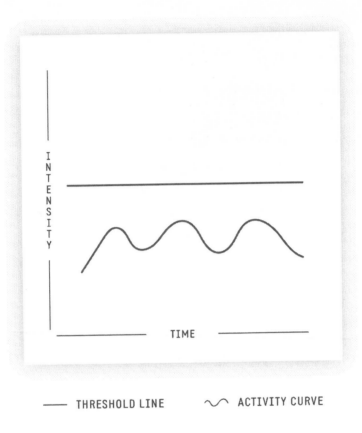

_____ THRESHOLD LINE   〜⌒ ACTIVITY CURVE

MSG: BASELINE

The above graph is a baseline model of the Movement Story Graph. The axes, depicted by the x- and y-lines, represent time and intensity, respectively. In this case, the horizontal line (x) measures time, while the vertical line (y) measures intensity. The x-axis can span any amount of time, depending on what activity, task, or sport you're measuring. It could be representative of the time it takes to do some light gardening, finish homework at your desk, mingle at a cocktail party, or go for a three-mile jog. Similarly, the y-axis can represent any unit that quantifies the level of exertion needed to perform whatever activity, task, or sport you're measuring on the x-axis.

The undulating line you see above the x-axis is your <u>activity</u> <u>curve</u>. For the sake of a simple explanation, let's pretend you chose a sixty-minute run as the activity you want to measure. The curved line, then, correlates the intensity of your run over the course of an hour. Meaning the x-axis represents zero to sixty minutes, and y-axis represents how hard your body works every minute.

So, in this example, you can imagine your run begins with a brisk, low intensity warm-up before increasing the intensity slightly to a light jog after just a few minutes. As you come to some hills, the intensity increases on the inclines, as your muscles work harder to carry you up the hill. But as you come down the hills, you have an opportunity to recover a little and slow your pace before your run levels out and you begin cooling down. This pattern accounts for the rise and fall of the activity curve, or the increasing and decreasing intensity level, over time.

Not a runner? It doesn't matter. As I mentioned earlier, your activity curve can measure the time and intensity of literally *any* activity. That includes standing for a few hours at an office party, struggling through the morning boot camp class your friend dragged you to, or even doing next-to-nothing for several hours during a lazy Sunday. Whatever you're doing, the activity curve represents the movements you do in any given timeframe that may be related to your pain.

At this point your pain is the only thing we haven't yet mapped on your MSG, but it is there. On your MSG, your pain is depicted by the horizontal line that rests above the activity curve and intersects the y-axis. This is called your <u>threshold line</u>. Your threshold line represents your <u>bandwidth</u>, or your body's physical capacity to handle the sustained intensity of each activity. In this regard, your threshold measures your body's physical limit, or the level of intensity your body can handle before it exhausts itself or, worse, breaks down.

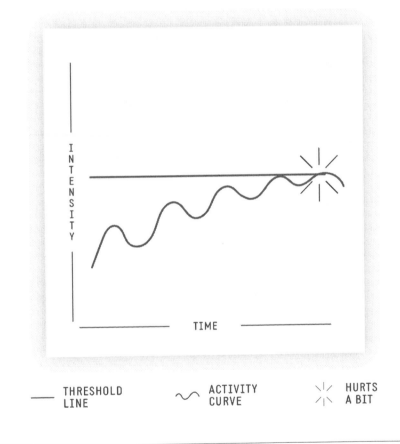

THRESHOLD LINE   ACTIVITY CURVE   HURTS A BIT

MSG: HITTING THRESHOLD

In terms of the MSG, exhausting your bandwidth equates to seeing the activity curve banging up against the physical threshold line, if not crossing it. As the lines meet, you might begin to experience a small sense of pain. Not yet serious, it's more of a burning or aching feeling that indicates some limit is being tested, some bodily system is being challenged.

Depending on your motive, you may come to crave that feeling, that release of endorphins, that high that comes from pushing your threshold. Some people become addicted to the rush of raising the bar, whereas some people prefer not to challenge themselves. They might shy away from a high-intensity class or avoid a trade show that requires hours of standing.

Either way, when your threshold is being tested, you have a choice: to keep pushing through it or to simply back off. Eventually we all back off; we stop the class, we go home, we rest. We put our feet up and allow our bodies to recuperate before we start a new day, a new class, a new project.

With the wide array of group classes or live-stream workouts available these days, you have an opportunity to take your favorite class practically wherever and whenever you want. In addition, social networks connect like-minded people who are chasing similar goals, pitting them against one another to see who can burn the most calories, put up the most reps, or run the most miles—all displayed on a scoreboard for the rest of the class to see.

While these types of challenges can encourage better fitness, there are downfalls, too. Because they're designed to test how close you can get to your threshold, how high you can raise the bar, or how much you can achieve compared to everyone else, there can come times when the risk of injury is overlooked in favor of progress. It's all too easy for participants to push through uncomfortable movements, muscle strains, and joint pains to stay at the top of the class.

Often, the primary cause of injuries in this case is repetition. As previously mentioned before, what happens to your muscles or joints in this situation isn't much different from what might happen to a paperclip under pressure. Imagine yourself at your desk, in class or at work, absentmindedly playing with a paperclip. You open it up and start bending it, back and forth, back and forth. After doing this for several minutes, you're brought back to reality as the clip snaps. Every time you bent it, the metal wore out a little more, becoming thinner and thinner.

Eventually the physical properties of the metal in the paperclip become increasingly malleable, losing stiffness and resistance as a result of the stress you repeatedly placed on it. On some level, the same thing happens to the tissues in your body when you apply excessive or repeated force; eventually the activity reaches an intensity that your body can't handle, you hit your threshold, and something snaps, causing you pain.

To make it more realistic, let's go back to the running example. If you only ever trained to run five miles, your threshold would be much lower than someone who has trained to run twenty miles. Surely you can imagine that if you tried to run more than five miles without stopping, you would likely exhaust yourself well before that 20th mile. Not only would you be out of breath, you might also have some sort of muscle injury in your calf, hamstring, or back. These are all indications that your activity (curve) has surpassed your threshold (line).

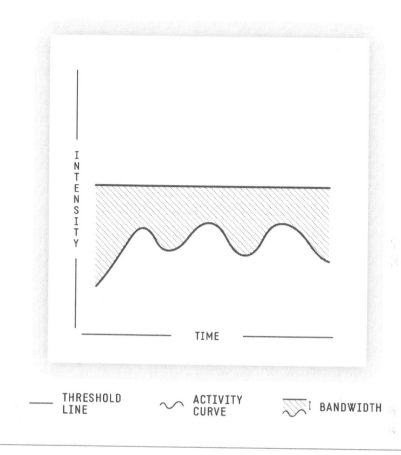

THRESHOLD
LINE   ACTIVITY
CURVE   BANDWIDTH

MSG: BASELINE ADD BANDWIDTH

That means the room you have to exercise or perform daily activities without pain exists in the space between your activity curve (the undulating line) and your threshold line (the horizontal ceiling). This capacity is marked in the graph above by the shaded area that is between the threshold line and activity curve. I refer to this space as your body's bandwidth. By definition, bandwidth technically refers to the amount of data that can be carried by a communication channel. But in terms of your body, your bandwidth is your ability to do an activity before reaching your threshold. It's essentially the range of capability you have, or the physical energy reserves you can rely on, to complete a sport or activity before becoming exhausted or injured.

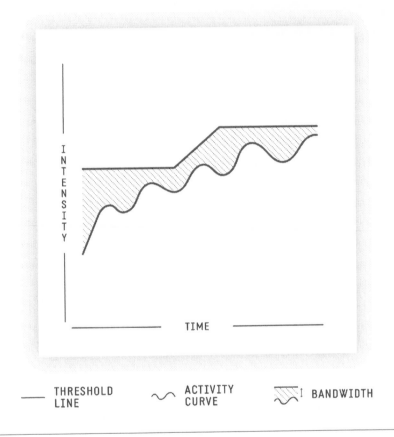

THRESHOLD LINE ⁀ ACTIVITY CURVE ▨ BANDWIDTH

MSG: RAISING THRESHOLD / MAXIMIZING BANDWIDTH

Of course there are activities that don't necessarily require us to exhaust ourselves, but it's human nature to test ourselves,[5] to push ourselves by varying degrees, to see just how much we can handle, to effectively raise our threshold and accomplish more. Like our individual lives, this desire to stretch takes many forms. We may challenge ourselves intellectually by learning something new, or physically through cardiovascular training or bodybuilding, or simply by doing our everyday chores.

Depending on your own spirit, and your underlying motives, you may be more inclined to keep testing your physical limits, even after you've hit your threshold. You tell yourself you can do just a little bit more, and then just a little more, and so on. When you're in this mindset, you're essentially trying to raise your threshold and influence how much your body can handle. If you do this carefully, you should be able to actually raise your physical threshold line and increase the bandwidth on your MSG.

I believe we all have an innate desire to not only reach our limits, but to create new standards and raise the expectations of ourselves. As we train properly, we can improve our strength, our speed, and our endurance, only to set a new goal, to continue raising the bar. But in order to more safely push yourself, physically and mentally, without causing distress, it helps to first identify where your physical and mental thresholds lie.

If we know we have more left in the tank we can intelligently test our bandwidth as we inch toward our limits. Let's think about it in real-life terms. Think about what you're working on right now, at home, at work, at the gym. Can you visualize any gaps you're trying to close? How are you currently trying to test your bandwidth? What activities require you to push it a little farther than you would normally?

Maybe you're on a tight deadline at work that's keeping you at the office for longer hours. Maybe you're training for a marathon that's coming up soon and you have to start running longer or faster, or both, to get ready for the race. Or maybe your friend talked you into a week of unlimited hot yoga, and you've been inspired to reach the same intricate poses that some of the other yogis do with apparent ease. These are all ways in which we test our personal limits.

In most cases you have one of two choices: back down or push yourself. If you're reading this, I'm willing to bet you're the type who buckles down and says, "I got this." You get to work a little earlier, you run an extra mile, or you reach a little farther with your fingertips. Every time you go just a little bit further, testing and stretching your bandwidth, getting closer and closer to your threshold.

Whatever goal you're chasing, your MSG helps you visualize your current capabilities. Of course, when applied to individual lives, everyone's Movement Story will have its own unique characteristics. Yet the overall principles will still reveal the distinct interaction between movement and pain that we encounter during the specific activities, sports, or tasks in our lives.

The Start of Pain and the Role of Inflammation

Now that you understand how to map your bandwidth, let's explore how even a minor injury can influence your threshold. We'll start with a common example: the ankle sprain. According to the American Orthopedic Foot & Ankle Society,[5] 25,000 people sprain an ankle in the U.S. every single day. Because so many people experience this injury, an ankle sprain can help you understand what pain is, what reactions take place within your body, and what changes occur as you return to normal.

In a nutshell, when your foot hits something unexpected—like a curb or another person—the muscles, ligaments, and other fibers that help support and protect your ankle don't have time to brace themselves for the load. That's why your ankle buckles. The swelling that comes next is your body's inflammatory response, a reaction that tries to protect the joint from further damage. It's also an obvious sign that something is wrong. So, while swelling can seem like a bad thing, it's actually your body's way of defending itself.

The inflammation itself is a physiological reaction caused by chemical mediators in your body. Chemical mediators, sometimes referred to as neurotransmitters, are chemical substances your body produces and sends to your nerves, muscles, or glands whenever necessary. When it comes to inflammation, the most notable chemical substances your body produces include substance P, CGRP, interleukins -2, -4, -6, and other histamines.

Eventually, the amount of chemical mediators reaches a tipping point, setting off what's known as an <u>action potential</u>—a spike in electrical activity caused when a neuron in your brain sends information down an <u>axon</u>, the long thread-like part of a nerve cell, to other cells. The action potential is launched by a receptor in your body called a <u>nociceptor</u>, or a special <u>sensory neuron</u>, which responds to potentially damaging stimuli by sending warning signals to the spinal cord and the brain. Finally, the nociceptor, the fiber that receives the influx of inflammation <u>mediators</u>, acts as a gatekeeper of the way pain is generated and perceived.

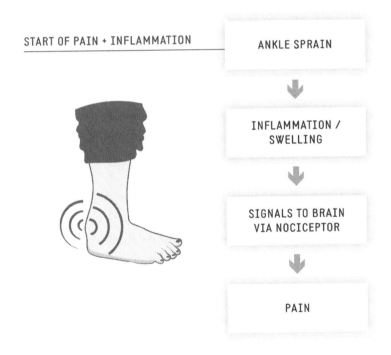

START OF PAIN + INFLAMMATION

ANKLE SPRAIN

INFLAMMATION / SWELLING

SIGNALS TO BRAIN VIA NOCICEPTOR

PAIN

Once your threshold has been met or exceeded, the action potential occurs and the nociceptors send a signal from your sprained ankle, up your spinal cord, to tell your brain that something is wrong. We refer to this entire process as <u>peripheral sensitization</u>, or sensitization of the peripheral nociceptor, where peripheral refers to any nociceptor outside your spinal cord. Ultimately your brain receives the nociceptor signals—triggered by the action potential as a result of the chemical mediators—and tells you that you're in pain.

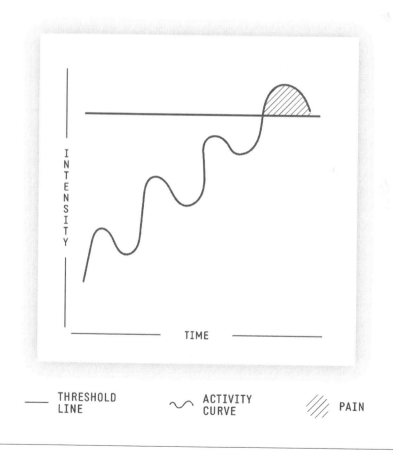

| THRESHOLD LINE | ACTIVITY CURVE | PAIN |

MSG: PAST THRESHOLD - PAIN

In the case of a sprain, your ankle, as well as the ligaments and tendons surrounding it, undergo sudden and unexpected stress. In response, inflammation swells the joint, the nociceptive fibers receive the inflammation signals, and your brain tells you it hurts. That, in essence, is the most basic form of peripheral sensitization, or the process through which an injury causes inflammation and pain. You can understand that all of this takes place after your activity curve surpasses your physical threshold line, meaning your body has no bandwidth to handle the physical load you're placing on it. The inflammatory response then sets off an action potential, causing peripheral sensitization of the nociceptor and alerting you to the pain.

These basic principles of injury, inflammation, and sensitization apply to any tissue in your body, and the same process occurs for essentially every injury, including muscle strains, herniated discs, or other compromised structures. Understanding this process that causes pain will help us understand what happens next, after the initial pain subsides.

In the same way it automatically responds to injuries, your body also has a natural way of healing itself. In most cases, your body will respond to the inflammation by sending white blood cells, immune cells, hormones, and nutrients to help heal the injury. As these cells work to reduce the inflammation, begin healing the tissue, and return mobility to your ankle, the chemical mediators decrease and the nociceptor cells receive fewer signals, quieting the warning that tells your brain you're hurt. Eventually the pain goes away altogether, and you start moving on it again, all the while assuming everything is all right and your ankle is perfectly functional again.

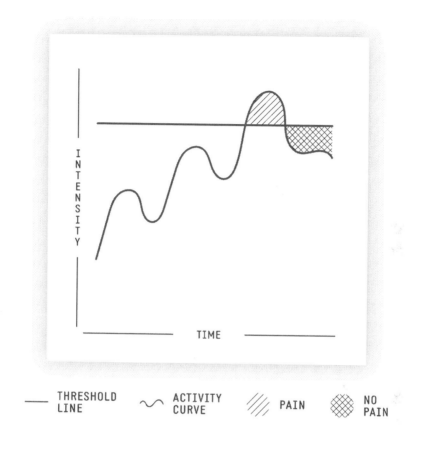

THRESHOLD — LINE   ∿ ACTIVITY CURVE   ⧄ PAIN   ⧆ NO PAIN

MSG: BELOW THRESHOLD - NO PAIN

The problem is that oftentimes, it's not. Especially with cases of unresolved pain, what we find is that the activity curve no longer drops below the threshold line.

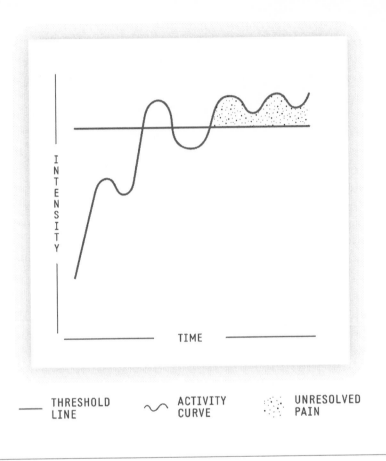

THRESHOLD LINE   ⌒ ACTIVITY CURVE   ⋰⋱ UNRESOLVED PAIN

MSG: UNRESOLVED PAIN

Whether it be ongoing pain from an ankle sprain, persisting lower back pain, or another area of your body that continues to hurt, my guess is that the graph above is the one that most closely resembles how you feel. That's because your body's bandwidth to handle more physical load, emotional stress, and other factors you may have previously been able to handle has been depleted.

Instead, you now maintain a state of pain that you won't be able to relieve until you determine which major factors have pushed you past your threshold.

This is why understanding the context around your pain narrative is vital. One by one, they become contributing factors that cause you to go above and beyond your threshold. Conversely, as you work on addressing the factors that shape your pain story, you'll be more equipped to start healing properly and relieve the unresolved pain you've been dealing with.

To help you explore your own pain narrative, we'll apply the previous components of who, what, where, when, and how to help you complete your own Movement Story. Remember that your graph may take time to complete. Later, we'll also incorporate the details about your body's natural design, which is much more objective in describing how the human body works, especially when it comes to pain. As we continue, we'll apply the principles of design to your Movement Story, and, piece by piece, you'll begin to see the big picture of your unresolved pain.

Creating Your Own Movement Story

Starting with the information we already have, let's refer back to the notion that a picture is worth a thousand words and visualize your MSG that helps you get a complete picture of your unresolved pain.

Now, regardless of the type of pain you're dealing with, the location, or the cause, there's usually a marker, or moment in time, you can recall when the pain manifested itself into something that really began to affect you and simply would not go away.

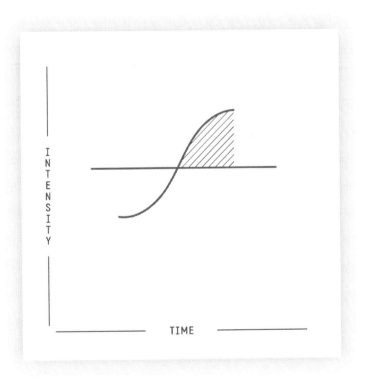

 PAIN

For practical purposes, I'd encourage you to use that moment as your starting point. Even if it's not the reason your pain began, it can serve as a benchmark we can build upon. That means that moment on your MSG would indicate where your activity curve first goes past your threshold line and does not go back below it.

You may have had other pain or injuries that caused your activity curve to spike and then return below the threshold line as the pain got better with rest or intervention—those should not be included. For the exercise, I want you to think only about the moment you noticed your pain continued to linger or persist even after it had recovered so many times before; this marker should indicate the moment your pain no longer healed.

If you used your pain narrative for reference, your graph would start with your primary pain complaint. It should be the pain that stopped you from doing what you enjoy for long enough to make you want to see someone about it. Beyond that, it should represent a pain that other health practitioners have attempted to diagnose and treat, but have not been able to or, worse, have wound up causing you more pain. It's the moment that led to where you are now, with your activity curve sustaining itself above your threshold line, where you're frustrated by an inability to find the answers you're looking for. You might feel depressed or hopeless at the thought that you might have to live with this pain for the rest of your life.

But like Diane, who experienced the myopic views within the healthcare system that could not see the bigger picture, you've reached the point where you must step back to see your story in greater context. Rather than looking at your injury from a structural orthopedic perspective, such as having arthritis or degenerative disc disease, think about it more comprehensively. Let's start tracing your activity curve backward from your primary pain complaint to see what factors may have caused or triggered your pain in the first place.

Example: Three Unique Scenarios for Sam

Let's use an example to help you understand how common pain symptoms can be traced back to different causes, and thus lead to different diagnoses. Let's get to know someone we'll call Sam, who has chronic low back pain and was diagnosed with degenerative disc or joint disease in the lumbar vertebrae. Sam's physician basically said: "You have degeneration in your spine. That's why you have chronic low back pain, and it can't be fixed because it's already degenerated. We can treat it with medication, injections, or surgery that may provide relief, but ultimately it will never heal because it's just too worn out."

In this case, this is the moment in time when Sam's low-back pain became chronic and persistent; this is the primary pain complaint where the activity curve continued to stay above the threshold line. But, as with the case of Diane, Sam's diagnosing doctor never asked Sam about the who-what-where-when-how details. The physician never looked to define the story that led Sam to chronic back pain. Or, in terms of his MSG, neither Sam nor the physician took time to trace the curve backwards or give context to why the pain went past the threshold.

Why does it matter if the doctor said there's nothing they can do about the degeneration in Sam's back? Well, let's explore three different scenarios with more context about who Sam is. Then let's see if that information changes how you view the spine degeneration and whether you think it's really the cause of Sam's low-back pain. In each scenario, try to think about how the activity curves might look different, even as they all end up going past the threshold line.

Scenario 1: Sam, The DIY Pharmacist

For the first scenario, let's imagine Sam is a pharmacist who stands for eight to ten hours a day, counting pills and filling prescriptions for his patients. For the last twenty-five years, he stayed on his feet to get the job done and he rarely sat down, as he and his wife had four children they supported financially and put through school.

Through the years, Sam's back would ache intermittently, but he noticed his pain was more intense at the end of the workday and even more so at the end of the week. Sam would also experience massive flare-ups on the weekends, as he would focus on taking care of all the do-it-yourself (DIY) chores that had to be done. When these chores included things like bending over to pull weeds in the backyard or getting into the bathtub to change part of the faucet, he would have intense back pain episodes. It was so intense that he would have to lie in bed for the rest of the weekend to recover. By Monday morning, he would have to toughen up so he could get back to work and resume standing all day.

Finally, five years ago his pain became more persistent throughout the day and during the entire week. As he became very vulnerable to increasingly intense and constant back pain, he could no longer pull weeds or handle chores that required much bending or lifting. He simply now had a tough time just getting through a normal day.

Scenario 2: Sam, the Former Football Player

Now let's say Sam is a thirty-year-old male who has had chronic back pain for the last fifteen years. Of course, that is a young age to experience chronic back pain, and his doctors would say the X-rays of his low back looked like those from a seventy-year-old arthritic man. How can that be?

Well, in this case, Sam would say it all started when he played high school football in his hometown. He was one of the bigger guys on the team, so there was an expectation for him to be one of the strongest as well. But because his school didn't have many resources, the team worked out in an archaic weight room and their strength and conditioning coach, who had been the trainer for thirty years, still used old-school lifting principles.

Because of the expectations placed on Sam to be a strong lineman, the strength coach homed in on him. While form and mechanics were not the coach's concern, he instead focused on repetitions, weight, and maxing out Sam's ability to lift. Because of that, Sam suffered a fracture in his lumbar spine, or a pars defect, at the age of sixteen.

Unfortunately, a pars defect is a common injury in adolescents who play sports that require a lot of back extension (or bending backwards), including cheerleaders, gymnasts, volleyball players, or simply weightlifters. The problem is that there's no surgery that can repair a pars defect, and usually a doctor can only recommend rest and recovery to allow the fracture to heal.

While Sam did his best to rest, he also tried to play and lift despite his pars defect until he eventually gave up football in high school. As he focused on his collegiate and graduate school education, his studying required him to sit all day long. And even though he was not lifting or playing football anymore, he found that sitting for his studies was actually more difficult and more painful than playing football. Still, he mustered through it.

By the time he was thirty, his back pain had become constant and unbearable, yet all his doctors said there was only so much they could do because of his severe degeneration. He received injections for short-term relief and even had surgery to remove a herniated disc, but nothing ever gave him the complete relief he hoped for.

Scenario 3: Sam, the Postpartum Mom

This time, let's imagine Sam is a woman. At forty-five years old, she has had chronic back pain for the last ten years. Her doctors said her degenerative back problems were hereditary and came from her parents. The doctor jokingly told her, "You picked your parents incorrectly," in an attempt to make light of the situation.

While she considered injections, medications, and surgical options, they never seemed like the best solution because the degeneration in her spine was not as severe as the example in the previous scenario. And even though her degeneration was more marginal, the doctors still couldn't figure out why Sam's back pain was so intense or see any other reason why it hurt.

They tagged her with a blanket diagnosis of degenerative joint disease in her low back, but what they missed was that she was a stay-at-home mother of three children. Furthermore, she had experience hard, laborious deliveries with the first two children, who were born through natural vaginal deliveries that made her determined to push the babies out. By the time she was ready to have her third child, there was so much pelvic-floor damage from her first two deliveries that the doctors required her to have a cesarean delivery, or C-Section.

She also found that she almost always had to carry one of her children on her hip while she made lunch or dinner or talked on the phone. With three young children and a house to take care of, she had no time to exercise. Although her husband was supportive, his help was limited to weekends when he was not working.

Through it all, by the time Sam turned thirty-five years old, her back pain became so intense it was almost unbearable to carry and take care of her three kids. But she was a tough-as-nails person who saw no room for a break, so she simply continued to fight through it.

Three Different Diagnoses

In the first scenario, I would say Sam the Pharmacist has degenerative back pain as a result of being on his feet way too long. His career and commitment to paying the bills essentially caused muscle fatigue in his legs and back, as well as extensive compression in his low back. In terms of his 24-hour pattern, his pain was initially more noticeable at the end of the day and especially at the end of the week.

But the fact that he had larger blow-outs with back pain on the weekends, when he had DIY tasks that required bending over, is important. After standing all week and fatiguing himself, getting down in a fully bent position all of a sudden caused too much disparity in his activity level, making him more susceptible to injury. The repetition of standing all week and then randomly lifting caused too much wear and tear on his back, and led to his degeneration.

In this scenario, Sam's Movement Story would show an activity curve that led up to the point where he had debilitating back pain based upon twenty-five years of accumulation from standing all week. The curve would show spikes of pain that indicated his bandwidth was moving closer and closer to the threshold line because he had no more capacity to stay on his feet or pull another weed after doing it for twenty-five arduous years. Finally, for the last five years, his pain became constant and persistent. This is shown on his activity curve as the line stays above his threshold line.

But what would have happened if Sam the Pharmacist had taken better care of himself during those twenty-five years? What if he had simply taken breaks and had not stood for eight to ten hours straight? What if he had taken time to get his leg muscles and core muscles stronger, allowing his muscles to last longer throughout the day? What if he had received help fixing things around the house instead of trying to do it himself?

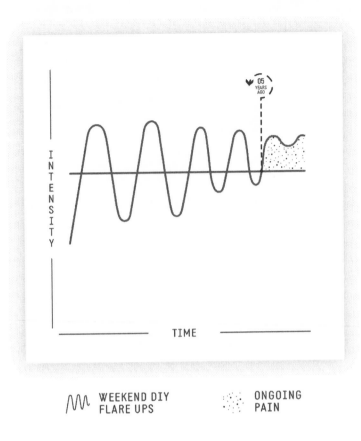

WEEKEND DIY FLARE UPS

ONGOING PAIN

MSG: SAM 1 - DIY PHARMACIST

I'd guess that if he had done any of those things, Sam the Pharmacist would probably not have been in so much pain, his doctors wouldn't be so quick to say it was caused by degeneration, his activity curve wouldn't come so close to his threshold line, and he would have more bandwidth between flare-ups. This is why it's important to see Sam's pain in the context of his lifestyle and not just by focusing on his X-ray results.

When it comes to the second scenario with Football-Star Sam, I would have to question why a thirty-year-old has the back degeneration of a seventy-year-old. Sure, it's possible there's a genetic component, but in reading through his case we can see that his wear and tear was accelerated by extraneous weightlifting and playing football. It caused so much damage that it led to the development of a pars defect at just sixteen years old. After that, the sustained pressure on his back from prolonged sitting for his studies in college and graduate school only made it worse.

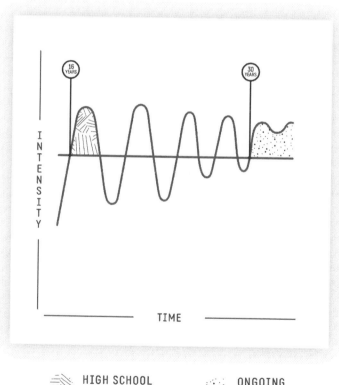

HIGH SCHOOL
LIFTING INJURY

ONGOING
PAIN

MSG: SAM 2 - FORMER FOOTBALL PLAYER

Of course, he would have been better off if he hadn't played football or if he'd at least been taught to lift weights correctly. But even so, the better question to ask is what would have happened if Sam had been taught to use his core and back muscles properly, even after he suffered the pars defect? What if he were taught to take breaks and stretch every hour instead of sitting for ten hours straight to study?

In my opinion, all these measures could have improved the mechanics in his back, decreased the intensity of his pain, and potentially slowed the degeneration in his spine. In fact, Football-Star Sam was a real patient of mine, and teaching him these things did relieve his pain. In his case, and in many others, proper education about why his back hurt and how it came about proved to be a more powerful form of intervention than any injections, medication, or surgery.

In our final scenario we have Sam the Mom. It's important to note that if your doctor says, "Your symptoms don't match what the test findings indicate," you can take it as a clue to look elsewhere. In this case, Sam the Mom's degeneration was not as severe as the doctors thought, just based upon the intensity of her pain. This is because her back pain was not from wear and tear, but rather from a lack of muscle control in her trunk and pelvis.

After having two pelvic-floor tears and an abdominal incision to deliver her babies, she was essentially left with no muscular stability around her trunk and pelvis. But after having healthy babies, her obstetrician gave her a clean bill of health and Sam resumed her role as a stay-at-home mom. No one directly encouraged her to regain her muscle tone after bearing children and she had little time to do so anyway, especially with her husband traveling.

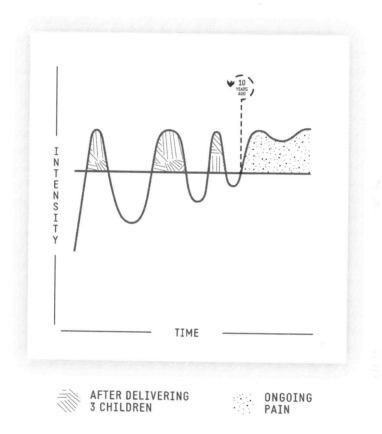

AFTER DELIVERING
3 CHILDREN

ONGOING
PAIN

MSG: SAM 3 – POSTPARTUM MOM

But do you really think she simply picked her parents incorrectly or that her genetics were to blame for her back pain? Or do you think it had more to do with having all the muscles around her trunk and pelvis torn or cut and putting her body back to work without proper rehabilitation? Could her pain have been compounded by standing, lifting, and carrying her children wherever she went? Do you think her degenerative back pain came out of the blue, or can you see how the previous events led up to her unresolved back pain?

It makes sense now that in any of these scenarios, the primary pain complaint of our "Sams" depicted on their Movement Stories would be a result of overuse that caused the so-called paperclip to snap. In fact, each of these examples were based on patients who were confused because they believed their back pain was truly related to structural degeneration of the spine. None of them ever considered the context of who they were, the work they did, the sports they played, or that, over time, seemingly harmless activities could lead to back pain.

In the end, having the context of their entire story gave them more insight and information about their persistent back pain than any X-ray, scan, or medical diagnosis could have provided. It was with that context, paired with the body mechanics we'll discuss in the next section, that I was able to identify the cause of their unresolved pain and ultimately provide a chance for them to heal.

Reflecting on Your Movement Story

Now that you've seen the importance of working backward from your primary pain complaint, let's go back to your Movement Story. Once again, think about your primary pain complaint as well as the pain or symptoms you're experiencing that have passed their threshold and left you feeling frustrated or depressed. Were you given a structural diagnosis that did not relieve your pain, even after intervention? If so, let's move backward.

Just like we did with the Sam scenarios, start looking back on your own pain story and ask yourself how you got hurt, and what previous activities could you have done that led up to the pain you feel now? (If you're not sure, don't worry. We'll explore the physical changes your body undergoes after injury in the next section.)

Remember to ask yourself what sports or activities you did or still do that could have provoked your pain. Did you do anything about it or did you just try to muscle through it? Was your pain accumulative or aggravated toward the end of the day or even the week?

As you ask these questions and trace your story back through the first section, can you start to see more reasons your pain has evolved to what it is now? Hopefully, you can at least appreciate how a single X-ray may not contain the entire explanation of your pain story.

Summarizing Your Pain Narrative

Now that we're coming to the end of this section, you should have taken the time to detail your own pain narrative, describe your symptoms, and incorporate the context of who you are. We've also introduced to you a visual tool known as the Movement Story Graph (MSG), which hopefully enables you to create both a timeline and a narrative that provides insight and captures your unresolved pain.

Before we move on, let's take a few moments to reflect on everything we've learned about your pain so far. As we start exploring the details of body mechanics, there are a few key questions that will be important to keep in mind, as they'll help you tie it all together. Based on everything you've recorded, ask yourself:

- What are two or three main reasons I might be in pain? (Do your best to come up with something that is different from a structural diagnosis you might have received from a physician.)

- What are two or three activities or injuries, whether traumatic, repetitive, or insidious, that I think might have led up to my development of unresolved pain?

- What are some measures I can take to start addressing the activities or positions that might be causing my unresolved pain?

Hopefully you have more clarity than you started with, but I'm guessing you also have a few more questions. That's why the next section will address the more objective part of your Movement Story, focusing on the body's design, especially as it pertains to pain. You can visit www.BrianYee.com for further resources to help you understand your narrative and how it relates to your unresolved pain, as well as ways to better conceptualize your Movement Story.

Further, as we discussed before, to fully understand your own Movement Story, you will need to keep reading the next section that will address the more objective part of your Movement Story, focusing on the body's design, especially as it pertains to pain. After that, we'll revisit your entire Movement Story to put it all together and identify next steps.

Like George Seurat's pointillism paintings, the work you've done thus far equates to the initial work of putting a few colorful dots on a large canvas. We'll keep adding details of your narrative throughout the rest of this book, so that by the end, you can take a step back and see the big picture of your unresolved pain unfold. For now, congratulate yourself on taking the time to reflect and establish vital components of your unique pain narrative. And remember to be patient as we move forward—the prospect of relieving your pain is just around the corner.

KEY POINTS TO REMEMBER:

- **Know your Movement Story Graph:** Your MSG is a visual representation that captures the timelines and the accumulation of different reasons why you experience unresolved pain.

- **Your pain is unique to you:** Your pain, in terms of intensity and location, may be the same as someone else's, but it will differ in terms of the cause of your pain.

- **Start from the beginning:** Understanding your unique reasons, characterized by your pain narrative, will start to give you clues for how to handle your unresolved pain.

PART TWO

How Pain and Injuries
Change Your Body

Section 2.1:

The Remnants of Pain and Injury

A s I've mentioned, your overarching Movement Story is broken into two equal parts: Your Pain Narrative and Your Body's Design. The first part, Your Pain Narrative, is essentially a subjective narrative that's unique to you, whereas the latter, Your Body's Design, is an objective, scientific perspective on the physiology of the body. Since we spent the first half of this book exploring Your Pain Narrative, the next half will be dedicated to Your Body's Design.

Let's think back to the example of the sprained ankle. Remember how inflammation and swelling could eventually turn into scar tissue? Similarly, the rest of the connective tissues intertwined throughout your body, which allow it to function, also have their own ways of dealing with injury, inflammation, and swelling.

Sometimes when injuries and inflammation occur, they can leave behind remnants, or traces of injury, throughout your body—and these remnants can affect the way you move in the future. More importantly, they can lead to a decreased ability for your body to properly function, and potentially put you at higher risk for pain and injury.

How the Remnants of Pain Impact Your Body

In this section, we'll explore common types of remnant changes that can occur in your body, as well as methods and interventions that can either fix or vastly improve these remnants. Just like an ankle with scar tissue, doing nothing to correct remnant changes will leave you with localized pain, limited movement, or a building block for pain elsewhere. By understanding the nature of these remnant changes you can identify and address them and restore yourself back to the natural design your body should freely have. In my experience, the following are the most common remnant changes that can occur in the body:

- Scar Tissue Formation
- Muscle Inhibition
- Myofascial Trigger Points
- Neurodynamics
- Fascia Restrictions
- Motor Control and Movement Pattern Changes

Scar Tissue Formation

One major change your body may undergo after an acute injury is the formation of <u>scar tissue</u>. In the most basic terms, scar tissue is a residual manifestation of the inflammation you develop following an injury. Essentially, your body creates fibers made of a protein called collagen to mend the tissue that has been damaged.[6] Unfortunately, the highly fibrous tissue doesn't handle tension well, nor does it offer the same structural support as a ligament, or have the ability to contract and elongate like a muscle. Unlike other connective tissues, scar tissue most closely resembles a cobweb; an intricate network of fibers that can limit the ability of a muscle to move freely.

In some cases, the development of scar tissue can be a greater concern for a surgeon than the injury itself. Especially for an orthopedic surgery like an ACL reconstruction or a hip replacement, there's a high risk of developing immobility after the surgery is performed. Why? Because after a surgeon cuts through your connective tissues to repair damage at the injury site, a large amount of inflammation occurs. (Remember, this is your body's natural response to trauma.) Unless the swelling is properly managed, these high amounts of inflammation can turn into excess scar tissue. So, although the surgeon may have repaired your ligament or replaced your joint, that success can be overshadowed if scar tissue formation inhibits your ability to move.

In the past, surgeons actually used to cast some orthopedic injuries for several weeks in order to stabilize the compromised ligament or joint. But over time, the inability to move the recovering ligament or joint gave the inflammation more time to develop scar tissue, ultimately reducing the mobility of whatever was repaired. Now orthopedic surgeons sometimes recommend physical therapy immediately after surgery, as long as it's safe. What they've found is that careful movement can help improve the integrity and stability of the connective tissues, providing longer-term support to their joint.

Remember, this doesn't apply to all injuries. Rotator cuff repairs, for example, need to be immobilized for a few weeks because the fragile nature of those tendons can be compromised if moved too quickly. In instances like that, the cost of losing the integrity of the repair is greater than the risk of scar tissue. This is one reason in particular it can be beneficial to coordinate with different kinds of doctors—like orthopedic surgeons and physical therapists—who work together to establish the best combination for moving, testing, and pushing a healing injury. Otherwise, missing that window can lead to immobility or cause re-injury.

How does this apply to an ankle sprain or other common injuries? Well, just like a knee that recently underwent surgery, a swollen ankle can also lose mobility from scar tissue formation if you don't know exactly when to rest it and when to move it. Even as the swelling dissipates and you feel like your bandwidth returns to normal, a layer of residual scar tissue forms around the ankle. You may not notice it, but that little layer can affect the mechanics of much more than your ankle—it can actually impact the way your whole body functions.

Basically, any build-up of scar tissue in your ankle will reduce mobility to some degree. This is also true of scar tissue anywhere in your body. As the scar tissue builds up, your ankle loses its ability to dorsiflex—or bend toward your shin—the way it would normally. Think about how you stand for a moment: at any given moment, your ankle joint acts as the junction between your foot and your upright leg. When standing, the angle between your foot and your leg is normally at 90 degrees. But because that's the <u>foundation</u>, we describe this position in joint mechanics as zero degrees of ankle dorsiflexion.

ANKLE DORSIFLEXION

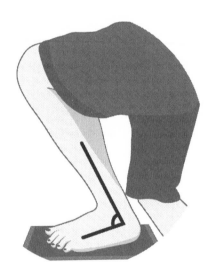

In the figure above, you will see the angle the ankle bends forwards called ankle dorsiflexion. Limitations in ankle dorsiflexion can make a difference in something as basic as walking, because when you walk, you put one foot in front of you to start the step and then push off the back foot to move forward. As your back foot and leg sweep behind you, you momentarily reach a point where your foot and ankle are directly underneath you, as though you are standing upright. Then, as your foot continues past your body, your ankle needs to dorsiflex 10 degrees to allow the rest of your leg to continue its stride.

While a healthy ankle bends a full 10 degrees whenever you walk, a sprained ankle may only bend 7 or 8 degrees, losing between 2 and 3 degrees of dorsiflexion overall. To you, the difference may be subtle. But with a sprained ankle, the heel of the injured foot leaves the ground earlier in the walking cycle, also known as a gait cycle, effectively altering every step you take. And although a few degrees don't seem like much, they can have a crucial impact when you walk 10,000 steps every day over your lifetime.

Worse, if you apply the same change in ankle mechanics to more strenuous activities, like running, squatting, or taking the stairs, the range of ankle dorsiflexion will exponentially decrease. Running, for example, requires 20 degrees of ankle dorsiflexion, while squatting and taking stairs require between 30 and 45 degrees of dorsiflexion, depending on how steep the stairs are or how low you can squat. With every more intensive activity, lacking a full range of motion in your ankle will have an even greater impact on your ability to perform effectively.

So even though your body has an amazing way of recovering from injuries and adapting to changes, at the end of the day it can only handle so much. Imagine someone who suffers from recurrent sprains or chronic ankle pain. Having sustained multiple sprains over time, a new injury may only take something as small as stepping on a pebble. Now it happens so often that you see it as a part of life, and you quickly brush it off, so much so that you don't even mention it when a physician asks about your injury history.

What you may not have realized, though, is that every injury led to a little more scar tissue formation and a little less dorsiflexion range. Worse, the change in ankle mechanics, however minimal, can have a greater impact on your body's natural symmetry. Because these changes don't just alter the way the ankle works, they can also influence the way other joints, like your knee and hip, work as well. And because your body's primary job is balance, decreasing your range of motion locally can also decrease your overall threshold, little by little.

As the presence of scar tissue increases with every injury and you endure decreased mobility or reduced muscle control, you may see the threshold line in your MSG decrease. Even though you feel normal, your previously injured joint is no longer working the way it used to, making it unable to handle the physical load placed on it. Even with just one ankle sprain, the threshold line decreases a little.

It may be so subtle that it goes unnoticed for a while. But with repeated injuries, your physical threshold line will decrease incrementally until the activity curve that would normally be within your limit now meets or exceeds your threshold during everyday activities. What this means is that the activities you once considered easy, like walking, running, or squatting, eventually become harder for you. As your bandwidth gradually decreases, you'll slowly but surely exceed your physical capacity earlier than you used to.

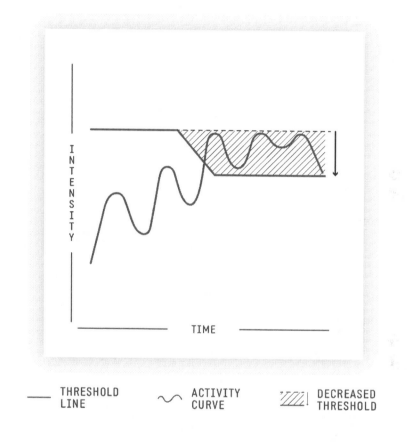

THRESHOLD LINE ACTIVITY CURVE DECREASED THRESHOLD

DECREASED THRESHOLD

Using the ankle example, it makes sense then that the first sprain would have to be caused by a large incident—missing a curb or landing on someone's foot—before you stumble to injury, whereas now, after having repeatedly sprained your ankle, it only takes something as small as uneven pavement to cause you pain. Or maybe it has begun to affect another body part that seems unrelated, like your hamstring. Maybe you used to run ten miles before your hamstring reached its threshold, but now you experience the same pain after just five miles. All because your overall capacity to handle the activity has been reduced over time.

How do we treat this? Well, when something swells, the first thing to do is try and reduce the swelling as quickly as possible by following four basic principles, commonly referred to as R.I.C.E.: Rest, Ice, Compression, and Elevation. In physical therapy, we can use hands-on techniques as well as recommend exercises to improve the mobility of the scarred down ankle joint. By performing specific exercises that improve the mobility of the scar tissue, the involved joint can then normalize its mechanics and function.

Muscle Inhibition

Muscles are the one connective tissue most people can identify because we can see them expanding and contracting as we move our arms and legs. We can also see how they get hurt after bumping into something and getting a bruise, or feeling sore the day after a hard workout. This type of pain, however, is usually considered to be a simple strain and not necessarily an injury that could cause remnant changes.

An injury is more likely to occur when you lift a box awkwardly and throw out your back, when you're involved in a car accident and your neck muscles spasm from the whiplash, or when you play too many games of pick-up basketball at the gym and you sprain your knee so bad it swells on the drive home. But what happened to the muscles in those injuries? Why didn't they work properly? Why do they hurt? And what happens to them after the initial injury?

Basically, the load that was placed on the muscles was more than they could handle. While in some cases your muscles can strain or even tear under pressure, sometimes significant injury can cause what's called *muscle inhibition.*

Muscle inhibition occurs when your muscles lose their connection to your cortical pathway, a nerve system in your brain responsible for muscle and joint function. Without this connection, the brain can't automatically decide when to activate your muscle. As a result, the muscle can lose some of its strength unless you do specific exercises to make sure it gets stimulated.

To be clear, though, muscle inhibition is not the same as muscle atrophy. In contrast, muscle atrophy refers to a loss of mass in your muscle specifically as a result of *underuse*—it has nothing to do with the neural connection to your muscles. Instead, you don't even have to be injured to experience muscle atrophy. This kind of muscle mass decrease can happen if you catch a bad cold or get busy at work and you simply haven't been able to work out for a week or two. Naturally, if you don't use your muscles regularly, they'll begin to shrink in size and tone. With atrophy, however, they'll return to normal as soon as you start using them again.

The same can't be said for muscle inhibition. With inhibition, your muscles are unlikely to quickly regain their strength even as you return to your normal activities. Because it's related to a broken connection to your brain, an inhibited muscle won't automatically get used once you start moving again. Instead, you'll have to specifically target the inhibited muscle to make sure it contracts properly and regains its mass.

For example, have you ever noticed the muscles in your thigh look smaller after spraining your knee? Or, ever injured your hip and noticed that your butt muscles don't look as full? If your muscles didn't bounce back once your injury healed, you likely experienced muscle inhibition. However, it can be hard to identify at first. That's because, unlike atrophy, muscle inhibition usually impacts the smaller, slow-twitch muscles closest to the joint rather than your larger, more obvious muscles. And since these are the muscles that stabilize your joints, instead of the ones that generate movement, they can go unnoticed.

Muscle inhibition can begin within 24 hours of injury, whereas atrophy would take weeks to develop. One study[7] in particular proved the immediate response of muscle inhibition following a low-back injury. It took just hours for the smallest muscles around the vertebrae, the lumbar multifidus muscles, to shrink in terms of their cross-section size. More importantly, the cross-section of the lumbar multifidus didn't automatically return to its usual size even as the pain receded and daily activities were resumed.

What that means is, if gone untreated, muscle inhibition can have a lasting impact on your body in two ways. The first is that as your muscle decreases in size, it starts an ongoing cycle of inhibition. Without direction from your brain, the muscle stops contracting, and continues to decrease in size. As it gets less and less use, the muscle can become so diminished that fat deposits begin to grow within the tissue, making it even harder to use. And what happens when those muscles stop doing their job? Your body finds a way to compensate, of course.

If your smaller muscles are unable to hold your joints together, your larger, fast-twitch muscles have to step in. And as they start to work overtime, holding your joints together *and* helping your body move, they fatigue faster. Worse, as your larger muscles exhaust themselves, they also exert more pressure and torque than your smaller muscles would, subjecting your joints to more wear as well. In turn, the joints above and below the injury now also have to step in to assist the body in movement. If, for example, you have a knee injury, and your quadriceps fatigue, your hip and ankle will also have to adapt to help you walk, squat, or run. This cascade of events can ultimately alter your body's most basic mechanics long after an injury occurs.

There are small muscles in your neck, known as deep neck flexors, that are also more likely to become inhibited after injury. Specifically, the longus colli muscle is a wafer-thin muscle that spans the entire front of your cervical or neck vertebrae. Along with the multifidus muscles on the back side of your cervical vertebrae, these muscles are designed to hold your head up in space.

People who suffered a whiplash injury can often experience fatigue or heaviness down the road. They commonly claim that their head feels so heavy by the end of the day it feels like they cannot even hold it up anymore. What they're describing is the inhibition of the deep neck flexors, the muscles that hold the cervical vertebrae upright. If this muscle group stops working properly, the joints lose a key stabilizing structure, making a normal thirteen-pound head feel more like a fifty-pound weight.

As a result, you can experience fatigue in your head or spasms and severe tightness in your neck as the larger neck muscles, like the scalenes and sternocleidomastoid muscles, work harder just to keep your head up. Other symptoms of inhibition in the neck muscles include headaches, nausea, and a change in spatial awareness. A lack of proper muscle support from the longus colli may even cause numbness or other nerve symptoms in your arm, as the cervical vertabrae can mildly compress against one another and irritate the nerves that extend to the arm.

Another place muscle inhibition can occur is in the gluteal or butt muscles, where it's commonly referred to as *Dead Butt Syndrome*.[8] Whenever I see a back or leg injury, one of the first things I ask the patient is whether they can contract, or squeeze, their butt muscles, first together and then one at a time. This is because when someone has an injury to their right leg, back, or hip, it will usually be much more difficult to contract the butt muscle on that side. You might even find, just by feeling the girth or size of the gluteal muscles, that they are smaller on the side of your injury.

When it comes to treatment, the problem with muscle inhibition is that you cannot simply lift weights and assume your inhibited muscles will automatically get activated again—that's only possible for muscular atrophy. Because muscle inhibition is an issue with the brain connection, it requires stimulating the muscle and getting it to contract in its natural sequence.

For example, if you found that one side of your butt muscles feels smaller than the other, try lying face down and raising one leg a few inches toward the ceiling. Without inhibition, you would normally feel your butt muscle engaging along with the back of your thigh and some of your back muscles; however, if your gluteal muscles are inhibited, when you raise your leg, you may not feel the glute muscle engage much. Instead you might feel a more significant contraction in your hamstring muscles at the back of your thigh, or even in your back muscles.

PRONE HIP EXTENSION

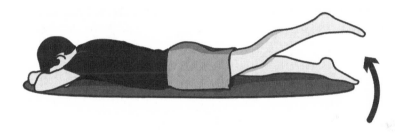

If you feel a cramp in your back or hamstring when raising your leg, it's an indication that those muscles are working harder than they should to compensate for inhibition in the glutes, which should be the primary muscles that contract. But if you start doing leg raises hoping to reduce the inhibition and get your glutes stronger, you may simply end up reinforcing a bad pattern. Without ensuring the proper sequence of the gluteal muscles, your hamstring and back muscles can become hypertrophied, or abnormally enlarged, causing secondary injuries in those areas, as the imbalanced muscles now dictate how you move.

What can you do about it then? Again, I'd recommend you work with a health practitioner who can help you re-engage any inhibited muscles. While there are many different strategies to help rehabilitate inhibited muscles, the idea behind the techniques should be specific and targeted toward helping your brain remember how to engage the muscle that has essentially lost its capacity to contract.

Once the muscle begins engaging again, you'll need to teach your body how to use it as part of the entire functional movement pattern of your body and integrate movements like squats, bends, or arm raises. You might be surprised to find that, once that pattern is set properly, you won't only feel less pain, but you might even feel stronger than you did before your injury.

Myofascial Trigger Points

Inhibition is not the only way your muscles can change after an injury. If you've ever had a massage therapist tell you that you have a lot of knots, you might have also wondered what those knots are. Maybe you imagined muscle fibers looping around each other like a pretzel or a shoestring, but that's not really what happens. Instead, what we call knots—areas that feel hard as rock but are tender to touch—are actually *myofascial trigger points*.[9]

What is a myofascial trigger point, and why can a little knot cause so much pain? More importantly, could a knot be at the root of your unresolved pain? Let's start with the definition: a trigger point is a hyperirritable spot in a taut band of skeletal muscle that's painful upon compression, stretch, overload, or contraction of the tissue, which usually responds with a referred pain that is perceived as distant from the spot.

What does that mean for someone dealing with unresolved pain? Once again, it serves as another reason you should consider the possibility that your pain may neither be coming from the exact place where your body hurts nor from a more traditional, structural source, like a herniated disc in your back, degeneration in your neck, or tendinitis in your shoulder. Rather consider that the muscle itself, surrounding your neck, back, shoulder, or wherever it may be, could be the primary reason you're experiencing pain, especially because myofascial trigger points can develop for a number of reasons.

They form most commonly when the muscle is traumatized in an abrupt event like a car accident, lifting injury, or sports injury. But they can also develop as a result of overuse and repetitive motions, meaning that simply overworking a muscle can cause myofascial trigger points. Another way they can form is through inflamed nerves. Just like a joint, nerves can become inflamed, though nerves can also send inflammation to the places where they terminate. Therefore, nerve inflammation can spread into a muscle, creating a myofascial trigger point.

The problem is that a myofascial trigger point is part of a chain of physiological changes that can cause referred pain elsewhere. For example, you might find that when you squeeze a myofascial trigger point on top of your shoulder muscles, you can feel pain radiate up to your head, causing ongoing or recurring headaches you might have had for years. Conversely, if you squeeze it without causing pain, you might find that it helps to diminish your headaches.

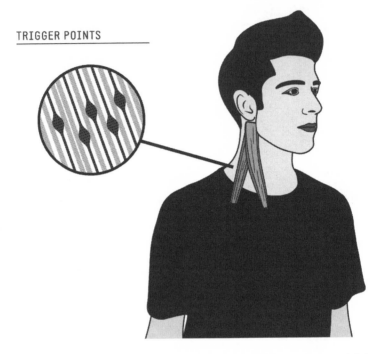

TRIGGER POINTS

Furthermore, inflammation can also occur within the myofascial trigger point itself. So the inflammatory mediators we discussed before, like substance P, CGRP, interleukins 2, 4 and 6, won't be found just in the swelling of an ankle sprain, but also within a related trigger point.[10] This inflammation creates a hypersensitivity and a taut band of muscle fiber, making it feel like a knot in the muscle.

Unfortunately, once myofascial trigger points form, they don't just go away on their own. Worse, they can become more problematic if they go untreated. That's because, in addition to causing your pain, myofascial trigger points can also change the way the muscle works. Having knots limits the muscle's capacity to elongate and develop proper contraction, and those changes alone can lead to other compensations or adaptations. For example, as the muscle stops doing its job, it can put a more abrupt force on the joint it moves or influences, causing injury to the joint, tendons, or ligaments. From there, small changes in the way one part moves can influence your body as a whole, effectively altering your entire movement pattern.

Sounds daunting, doesn't it? In many ways it is, but the good news is myofascial trigger points *can* be treated. The most common methods of treatment include massage, cold lasers, ultrasounds, and dry needling. Dry needling is a technique used by physical therapists specifically for muscles. In this treatment, we insert a dry needle, free of injections or medications, through the skin and into the muscle.

Dry needling targets <u>trigger points</u>, or tense areas of fascia and muscle, that are otherwise hard to reach by hand. As the needle reaches the myofascial trigger point, it elicits a response that releases inflammation from the trigger point, allowing it to heal and restoring the muscle to its normal operating capacity.[11] When appropriate, dry needling can be a highly effective technique to treat trigger points and their involvement in your unresolved pain.

Neurodynamics[12]

Other changes that take place within your connective tissues may affect your nervous system. When you think of nerve pain, you might think about paralysis, sciatica, or a spinal cord injury. But an important fact you might be unaware of is that your nerves are a connective tissue just like muscles or ligaments. In fact, nerves are one of a few systems that span the entire body. The only other tissues that really go from head to toe include your skin, fascia, arteries, and veins, while your muscles, joints, and ligaments only extend from one region in the body to another.

Peripheral nerves, specifically, also have the capacity to elongate, stretch, and compress even better than a muscle can. The structures around the peripheral nerve, called epineurium and perineurium, allow the nerve to have both an elastic capacity and an absorbent capacity that enables it to withstand many forces. But like every other connective tissue, your peripheral nerves also have a limit to what they can withstand, and you can test it yourself.

Use an arm that hasn't had any nerve injuries or symptoms; reach outward, slightly upward, and behind you. If you reach far enough outward, you'll probably feel your muscles stretch, and if you reach a little further, you'll probably start to feel pulling, numbness, or tingling in your fingertips or your hand. That sensation is a sign that you're nearing your nerves' elastic threshold.

On top of that, peripheral nerves can also be compressed, like a soft sponge. You can squish the nerve, but if you press hard enough or long enough, it will eventually start to react, causing tingling, pain, or burning symptoms. A classic example of this occurs when you hit the funny bone in your elbow and you can feel numbness and tingling all the way to your fourth and fifth fingers. It happens because the ulnar nerve, which runs through the inside of your elbow, gets compressed and causes paresthesias, or a tingling sensation, down your arm.

It may sound surprising, but nerve-related symptoms are frequently tied to unresolved pain complaints. Think about it: while localized muscular pain isn't typically cause for concern, you might be alarmed when your leg or arm starts to tingle, burn, or buzz. You can almost be sure a nerve is involved, and something is really wrong. That feeling indicates a nerve is becoming sensitized.

Just like peripheral sensitization, nerves too can become sensitized in what we call neurogenic sensitization. Just like the sprained ankle example, nerves can become inflamed—not just around the outside, but also within the nerve itself. Neurogenic inflammation like this can spread throughout the nerve as it courses from your spine to your legs or arms, going beyond the point the nerve was initially injured and sensitizing the entire nerve.

This is why spine surgeons are often convinced a herniated disc, which compresses your nerves, could be the sole reason pain is shooting down your leg. However, once the nerve itself becomes irritated and sensitized, even if the disc was the original source of your sciatica, you end up with a separate tissue system in its own inflamed state. So, although some people might feel better after having surgery to remove a herniated disc, many people will still complain of nerve symptoms down their leg. A surgeon may say it will go away with time, but that's not necessarily true if the nerve itself is still inflamed.

The same way scar tissue can accumulate after an acute ankle sprain, inflammation that builds up in the nerve can settle in, causing it to become less elastic and less mobile than it used to be, even as the nerve-like symptoms calm down. People who suffer these symptoms usually have a sense of tugging in their arm or leg that they feel they always want to stretch, but when they do, their pain either gets worse or aggravates residual nerve symptoms.

Another problem that arises with this type of nerve restriction is that it cannot be diagnosed through standard nerve exams, such as nerve conduction velocity tests. This is because the problem doesn't lie in the nerve's ability to conduct; the problem lies in its ability to elongate and withstand tensile or compressive forces. So, while a nerve conduction test can be valuable for diagnosing conditions like multiple sclerosis or neuropathies, it does not measure the way a nerve should elongate and move with your functional movement. There are, instead, hands-on techniques through which physical therapists can assess the quality of a nerve's mobility, especially when it becomes sensitized and less mobile. These techniques are known as *neurodynamics*. Founded by Michael Shacklock, an Australian physiotherapist with whom I've been honored to study, is a leader in the field of nerve dysfunction. He defines *neurodynamics* as "the clinical application of mechanics and physiology of the nervous system as they relate to each other and are integrated with musculoskeletal function."

What this means is that, in order to understand nerves within musculoskeletal movement and function, we need to know the mechanical properties of how nerves work as well as the physiology of how the nerves conduct. To get sensitized or mechanically restricted nerves moving again, Michael has developed manual, or hands-on techniques. These neurodynamic techniques help restore the elastic and tensile properties of nerves, just like techniques and exercises that get a stiff sprained ankle moving again.

I recommend proceeding with caution when it comes to the delicate nature of how nerves behave, and I'd encourage you to work with a specially trained therapist who understands how neurodynamics work. Many patients have come to me because they flared up trying to do neurodynamic exercises that they found on YouTube. They did not understand which one to do and ended up being too aggressive with them. The good news is that once you learn how to get the nerves to elongate and move normally again, your symptoms of tugging, tingling, and overall restriction will improve and your overall movement pattern can be restored to its natural state.

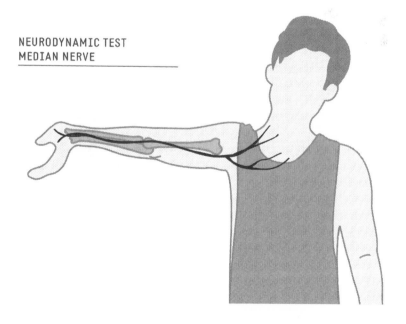

NEURODYNAMIC TEST
MEDIAN NERVE

Fascia

When you ask people what fascia[13] is, even though some have heard of it, most usually have no idea what it does. In layman's terms, you have fascia in your body that is a whitish, fibrous material between your muscles and skin. This is similar to the whitish material you see surrounding a piece of raw chicken meat when you prepare it for a meal. Just like the casing of a sausage link, fascia basically encapsulates the muscle and other connective tissues. However, fascia doesn't just surround your muscles; it's intertwined throughout your entire body. It exists throughout your internal organs, abdominal cavity, your nerves, and other connective tissues.

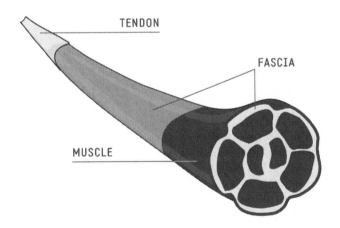

In general, the areas where fascia resides tend to be more dense. One of the densest and most broad areas of fascia can be found in the small of your back, in a structure called the thoracolumbar fascia. If you look at the anatomy of a human's back side, you'll see a broad whitish structure along the reddish muscles; that is your thoracolumbar fascia. Just like ligaments that support a joint, this area of fascia is a passive support structure designed to hold us up, especially when we sit and slouch.

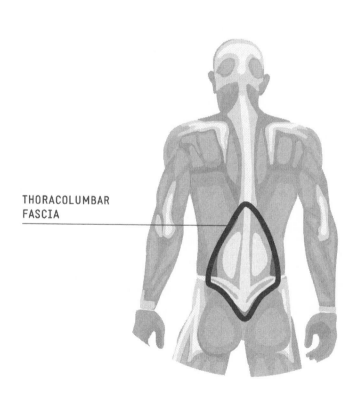

THORACOLUMBAR
FASCIA

The other thing this fascial structure does is help connect the adjoining muscles to make them work in sync with one another, like an energy transmitter. In reality, there are a lot of muscles that connect to the thoracolumbar fascia, including the gluteal muscles, abdominal muscles, and latissimus dorsi muscles. As one muscle group contracts to function, its force is transmitted through the fascia to create functional synergy as other muscles contract, allowing the rest of the body to move as you intended.

Have you ever noticed that when you walk, your arm swings forward as your opposite leg moves backward? This is known as a reciprocal gait pattern. The synchronicity of the opposite arm and leg moving in unison is achieved through the transmission of energy between the gluteal muscle and the opposite latissimus dorsi muscle, which are connected through the thoracolumbar fascia. Without this fascia, your opposite arm-leg coordination would be highly inefficient.

Just like with muscle and joint injuries, your fascia's connective tissue can also go through changes and maintain remnant effects when it becomes injured or inflamed. One of the key properties of fascia is that it's composed of a substance called hyaluronic acid. Hyaluronic acid allows the fascia to keep its fibrous state and still remain mobile, because in your everyday movement, you need fascia to be a supporting structure—not just a firm sheet that clamps down and keeps you from moving freely.

The problem is that when fascia is involved in your injury and pain, its hyaluronic acid becomes denatured, or depleted of its natural characteristics. The fascia then loses its mobility and elasticity as it becomes thicker and denser. Just like a myofascial trigger point, it can become a pain generator that causes changes to tissues or joints it envelops, and, just like inflamed or sensitized nerves can spread inflammation to your muscles and develop myofascial trigger points, your sympathetic nervous system can also send signals to your fascia. This process creates an inflammatory response that not only denatures the hyaluronic acid in your fascia, but can also leave the fascia in a compromised state that renders it unable to provide proper sensory feedback to your brain.

Fortunately, there are many clinicians and researchers dedicated to studying fascia[14] and how it relates to our everyday movement or pain,[15] as well as the techniques and interventions that improve its mobility. Like treating myofascial trigger points, manual techniques are an effective way to improve the mobility of your fascia. Fascial mobilization can be performed by a massage therapist, physical therapist, chiropractor, or athletic trainer, and there are even self-help devices, like massage rollers, vibration guns, trigger-point sticks, and pressure-point balls, that aim to improve fascial mobility. But it's important to first determine where the fascia is restricted and why it's happening.

Interestingly, some research suggests that your fascia is one of the main connective tissues that corresponds directly with your fight-or-flight system, also known as your sympathetic nervous system. This is the system responsible for the feeling you get when you hear a loud bang or an abrupt horn. The sensation may correspond with a sudden startle that makes you feel like a deer in headlights. In a trance, your eyes widen, hands and legs stiffen, and you feel a chill down your back. These sensations are a reflex stimulated by your sympathetic nervous system to brace you for an emergency.[16]

The sympathetic nervous system, which is part of your autonomic nervous system, also controls anxiety, depression, and other traumatic emotions. People with significant fascial involvement can also experience changes in their emotions or affect. They may be more depressed, anxious, or experience other extreme emotional responses. Surprisingly, when their fascia's mobility is improved using different techniques, many patients will feel nauseated or fatigued, and some even say they want to take a long nap. This occurs when the fight-or-flight system, which has been over-engaged, begins to relax and return to normal.

The counter system to your sympathetic nervous system is known as your parasympathetic nervous system. The parasympathetic nervous system is responsible for helping your body calm down, like hypnosis or meditation. In addition to restoring its connective tissue properties, improving the fascia's mobility can also help regulate the balance between the sympathetic and parasympathetic nervous system and re-stimulate hyaluronic acid in the tissue, restoring it to its normal functioning capacity. So, if you think you might be experiencing some type of fascial dysfunction, I'd recommend consulting a qualified health practitioner to discuss how your fascia might be involved in your unresolved pain.

Muscle Control, Movement Pattern Changes, and Pain

As a physical therapist, people typically see me because they have some sort of unresolved pain that affects their ability to move, function, or perform. But there are so many opportunities for the remnants of an injury to create changes, you might wonder how some people can move at all. Unfortunately, there are cases in which pain is so severe that it truly does stop them from moving, functioning, or playing a sport.

Why does this happen and how do we get your body working properly again? One of the main changes that occurs is an inability to use the proper sequence of muscles and joints that allows for efficient movement. We've also discussed structural changes to connective tissues, like scar tissue formation, cortical changes that inhibit muscles, trigger-point formations, reduced nerve elasticity, and loss of hyaluronic acid in fascia. But one of the most notable changes that takes place in our bodies following pain and injury is a change in the way we move!

As I've mentioned before, there are certain muscles that are designed to stabilize you and certain muscles that are designed to move you. This concept is known as local versus global muscle control. Local muscles comprised the smaller, slow-twitch, longer-lasting muscles located closer to a joint, while global muscles comprise larger, fast-acting muscles responsible for powering movement, force, and torque.[17]

One of the best examples of how these muscles differ can be

seen in your shoulder. Your rotator cuff muscles, for example, are the smaller, local muscles designed to simply hold your ball and socket joint together, while the larger, global shoulder girdle muscles, like the pectoralis or triceps, are designed to provide the power to lift, pull, or push in addition to offering stability. Notably, muscle inhibition occurs mostly to the smaller, local muscles, like the multifidus or longus colli muscles near the spine or the VMO muscle near the knee.

GLOBAL
MUSCLES

LOCAL / ROTATOR
CUFF MUSCLES

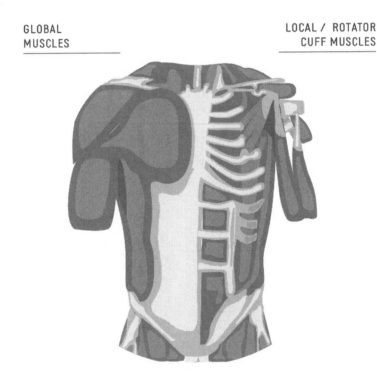

In addition to the differing roles of local versus global muscles, there is also another complementary way to look at how muscles play different roles in your body's daily function. A physician from

Prague named Vladimir Janda[18] looked at specific body regions and noticed muscle deficits. He was able to observe an entire body to see where certain muscles were inhibited and where others were overdeveloped, or hypertonic. Just by looking, he was able to determine where the patient's pain was located, how severe it was, and what their prognosis for recovery would be.

But rather than refer to them as local versus global muscles, Janda described muscles in two categories: tonic muscles and phasic muscles. Tonic muscles are considered the flexors, or the more dominant muscles involved in repetitive or rhythmic motions, while phasic muscles are considered the extensors, or the muscles that work eccentrically against the force of gravity. What Janda observed was that patients who experienced more chronic pain typically showed inhibition, or a decrease in the tone of their tonic muscles, while their phasic muscles appeared overdeveloped. Overdeveloped, however, does not mean they looked as though the patient went to the gym and lifted weights to get them bulkier. Instead, Janda noticed that the phasic muscles looked like they were almost in a state of spasm, as if bracing or guarding.

Similar to global muscles, the phasic muscles that were designed to provide larger movements were now also acting as compensatory muscles, doing the work of the tonic or stabilizing muscles that are meant to hold the body up. This disparity in muscle tone and compensation when it comes to simple support can be detrimental to the function of the body and can, by itself, be the core cause of your pain.

As an example, let's think back to the three scenarios with Sam.

Think about how Sam's tonic muscles, in the core, glutes, and deep neck, were unable to support the pharmacist while he stood all day, provide proper stability to the lumbar vertebrae when the jock lifted heavy weights, keep the mom balanced after giving birth to three children.

How much extra force was applied to the area where their local or tonic muscles are simply not as strong as they should be? When they fatigued and took a break, somehow the body figured out how to keep moving, keep achieving. To do that it calls on the larger, phasic muscles to take over. But without the counterbalance of the tonic muscles, the phasic muscle will apply more pressure, more torque, and more shearing forces to the joints, ligaments, and other connective tissues in the body. As a result, the adaptation can cause a series of events that leads to injury, inflammation, peripheral sensitization, and pain.

By understanding how different muscles play varying roles and how pain can make your muscles adapt and compensate based upon the state you are in, we need to take a more detailed approach in how exercises are prescribed and recommended. In my experience, exercises, whether they strengthen you or stretch you, are the things most people think they can do on their own. They can find their favorite class or training regimen virtually on their favorite app or class. For the most part, these can be very effective. However, once someone is dealing with ongoing pain, they now have muscle patterns that do not work the way they used to. By attempting the 'normal' regimens, people can often get hurt trying to do the 'right' thing. I find that many people dealing with unresolved pain issues are afraid to exercise because it hurts them more. If this describes you, it is vital that you find a qualified physical therapist that can properly assess your baseline muscle function and, more importantly, recommend the proper sequence and series of exercises that will restore the role of your local and global muscles, as well as re-engage the proper function of your tonic and phasic muscles. When you can establish this, you will feel like your body can move again more fluidly and with significantly less pain.

Nancy's Movement Story

To clearly show how an accumulation of remnant changes can serve as the building blocks of your unresolved pain, let's look at a patient case and define her Movement Story. Nancy was a thirty-five-year-old woman who complained of chronic back pain on her right side and achiness down her right leg. The pain started ten years earlier, when Nancy was moving furniture in graduate law school. While trying to lift an awkwardly sized and heavy sofa, she injured the right side of her back and felt a searing pain down the back of her right leg–a kind of pain she had never experienced before. At the time, she was diagnosed with a herniated disc in the right side of her lower back, at the L5-S1 level, and she received epidural steroidal injections that helped significantly reduce her pain.

However, she would still experience a residual soreness in the right side of her back and a sense of tingling or tugging along the back of her right leg. She would say it worsened or was aggravated with prolonged sedentary positions such as sitting as well as standing for more than twenty to thirty minutes. She also noted that she had some soreness while sleeping and felt mildly achy in the morning when she first woke up, but her pain would worsen as the day went on. There were days, after working long hours, that she would come home with searing pain down her right leg. While she knew that laying down briefly would give some relief, she did not have the time during work to do so.

NANCY'S PAIN NARRATIVE

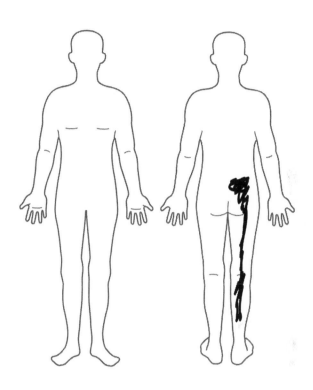

PRIMARY COMPLAINT:

RIGHT SIDED BACK PAIN AND ACHINESS IN RIGHT POSTERIOR LEG

MECHANISM OF INJURY

WHEN: 10 YEARS AGO
CATEGORY: TRAUMATIC
MECHANISM: LIFTING FURNITURE

NANCY'S PAIN PATTERNS

AGGRAVATING FACTORS:

AGGRAVATING ACTIVITY: PROLONG SITTING AND STANDING
TIME FRAME: 20-30 MINUTES

EASING FACTORS:

EASING ACTIVITY: LAYING DOWN
TIME FRAME: 15 MINUTES

24 HOUR PATTERN:

MORNING: MILDLY STIFF AND ACHY
EVENING: WORSE
NIGHTTIME / SLEEPING: OCCASIONAL SORENESS

Although Nancy had learned to deal with her ever-increasing symptoms over the years, her pain eventually became more persistent, and, because further epidural injections only helped a bit, doctors no longer thought the herniated disc was the cause of her pain. Nancy even tried physical therapy to improve her core abdominal strength, and saw a chiropractor for spinal adjustments, but neither gave her the relief she was hoping for. But as a high-powered attorney who regularly performed under stress, she felt she simply had to keep living life and push through.

It is something she learned from her high-ranking military officer father who told her that 'pain is for the weak!'

When Nancy came to my clinic, I took a thorough history in her first evaluation and discovered that she had been a high-level soccer player throughout her childhood, starting at the age of five. During those years, she sprained her right ankle numerous times, only to tape it up and get back on the field as soon as it could bear weight. During that time, she also suffered some hamstring strains as well as some mild hip pain on the right side. Still, she learned to fight through it and keep playing at a high level.

Later she said the pain she endured in soccer was nothing compared to the pain she experienced through college and law school. It perplexed her that her right hip would ache and pinch in the front, and her lower back would get tight and sore, even though she did nothing but sit in class or at the library. She figured it was just tightness, and the pain would go away like it had before. But when she lifted that heavy piece of furniture, her pain brought her to a halt. She was surprised that one piece of furniture would put her out of commission, after all the athletic things she had done in the past! She couldn't understand why, even with all the ankle sprains and other injuries she had, lifting a piece of furniture would be the injury that caused her the chronic pain that no procedures or interventions could fix.

NANCY'S PAIN HISTORY

MEDICAL / INJURY HISTORY

INJURY: MULTIPLE RIGHT ANKLE SPRAINS
WHEN: HIGH SCHOOL

INJURY: RIGHT HAMSTRING STRAIN
WHEN: HIGH SCHOOL

INJURY: RIGHT HIP PAIN
WHEN: GRADUATE SCHOOL

ACTIVITY HISTORY

ACTIVITY: COMPETITIVE SOCCER
DURATION: CHILDHOOD TO HIGH SCHOOL

ACTIVITY: GRADUATE LAW SCHOOL
DURATION: MID-20'S

ACTIVITY: OCCUPATION - ATTORNEY
DURATION: LATE 20'S TO CURRENT

MOTIVATING FACTORS

MOTIVATION: "PAIN IS FOR THE WEAK!"
SOURCE: MILITARY FATHER

How does Nancy's case translate to the context of what we have discussed so far? Well, let's start establishing a Movement Story perspective. Given Nancy's personal story and the remnant changes she incurred through past injuries, I would say that herniating a disc in her lower back in her mid-twenties was her tipping point. That means this would be the primary pain complaint where her unresolved or persisting pain began. Now, some ten years later, she has had ongoing pain that sustains itself above her threshold.

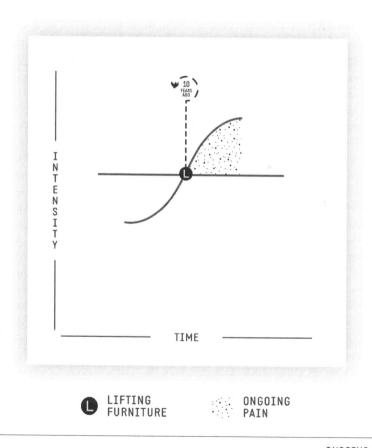

ONGOING PAIN

The problem is that her health practitioners spent ten years trying to treat her back pain and nerve symptoms because the location of her pain and her MRI results suggested she had a herniated disc. But from a Movement Story perspective, I would argue that the focus on where her symptoms were and what the MRI film showed was much too narrow. Instead we need to consider her entire story, including the remnant changes her body went through as a soccer player, a college student, and a non-stop career attorney.

As part of her pain narrative, we would need to include her ankle sprains in her previous medical history and consider soccer as a previous athletic activity that could influence the way her body functions now. For Nancy, the repetitive sprains to her right ankle while playing soccer set up a cycle of inflammation and scar tissue formation around her ankle joint. Because scar tissue can restrict the mobility of the area it surrounds, Nancy started to lose the ankle dorsiflexion required to run efficiently up and down the soccer field. The loss of ankle dorsiflexion in her right ankle caused Nancy to develop compensatory patterns that made the rest of her right leg function less efficiently. Without proper dorsiflexion, the hip socket and gluteal muscles cannot provide the power and stride necessary for running.

A result of the lacking hip function, Nancy developed muscle inhibition and myofascial trigger points in her right gluteal, or buttock, muscles. In her early twenties she noticed her hip right hip would ache from just sitting, and her hamstring would feel tight, because the muscle started to overwork to compensate for her reduced ankle mobility and the loss of muscle control in her hip. From there, we could see the back muscles on the same side start to work more. With this pattern, aches and strains in the back, which are essentially myofascial trigger points, are a common occurrence.

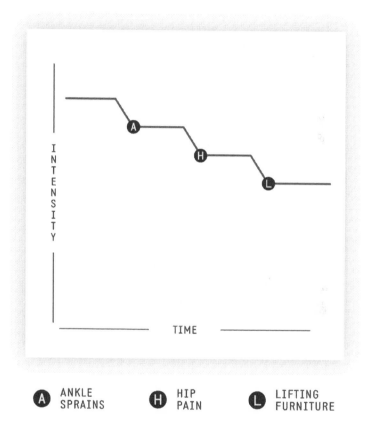

NANCY'S PAIN

Considering what we know about her Movement Story, do you think Nancy was in optimal condition to lift an awkwardly sized piece of furniture? With the lack of ankle mobility, muscle inhibition in her gluteal muscles, and myofascial trigger points in her gluteal and back muscles, Nancy had a limited bandwidth to handle the furniture. For years her activity curve reached closer and closer to her threshold. And even though she pushed through, training her body to raise her threshold and achieve more, eventually the remnant changes that accumulated caught up to her when she lifted the sofa. In that moment, her activity curve went past her threshold line and resulted in a herniated disc.

What may be most troubling is that there are cases in which an injection can fix a patient's pain. So why, in Nancy's case, did she suffer persistent pain for ten years? From my perspective, the herniated disc in her back caused her to develop nerve symptoms down her right leg, commonly known as sciatica. Although the epidural steroid injection helped calm the sciatica, Nancy likely had residual inflammation in her sciatic nerve. Eventually the nerve developed scar tissue that rendered it less mobile and less elastic. The sense of tugging or irritation in the back of her hip and leg was a sign that she maintained a level of neurogenic sensitization that kept her aware of it throughout the day.

Through her collegiate and legal studies, Nancy suddenly found herself sitting significantly more than she had in the past. The need to stabilize her in sustained studying positions was too much for her tonic, or local, muscles to handle, as her muscle control was altered from the injuries she had suffered in the past. That meant her larger, phasic muscles tightened more just to hold her up in a seated position, and her 24-hour pattern revealed she had more pain at the end of the day, as she sat for longer and longer periods. It was an indication that the muscle control providing enough endurance to last throughout the day fatigued earlier than expected.

In addition to carrying stress in her shoulder and back muscles, Nancy developed significant fascial restrictions through her thoracolumbar fascia and mid-back. This occurred as a result of compensation for the lack of proper muscle control and as a response to the fascia's connection to her fight-or-flight system, which controls stress and anxiety levels. In fact, Nancy never liked getting massages because these areas had become too sensitive to touch; it was such an unbearable experience that she simply avoided massages, even when she felt tight.

So even though the herniated disc may have pushed her pain past her threshold, it was all the remnant changes in her tissues and her movement patterns that made Nancy more vulnerable to herniating a disc. That's why an isolated diagnosis of a herniated disc and interventions to treat it ultimately had limited benefit. We also have to address the changes that occurred in her body after she herniated a disc in her back, such as the neural sensitivity and the elastic changes—not to mention the fascial sensitization and restrictions she developed as a result of reduced muscle control combined with her high-stress lifestyle.

Only when we see all these things together can we fully grasp the entire picture of her sustained, unresolved pain. Nancy's pain narrative is based on her injury history, the sports and prolonged activities she was involved with, and her accompanying pain complaints. Viewed together, her pain narrative, paired with the physiological changes, reveal an entire Movement Story rather than an isolated injury, like a herniated disc, sciatica, or degenerative disc disease. If we can view Nancy's Movement Story in broader context, it changes the way we would treat her unresolved pain.

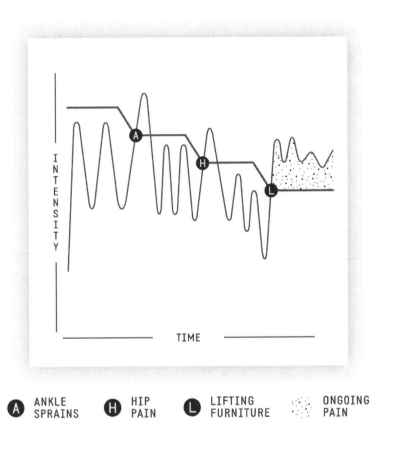

<table>
<tr><td>A</td><td>ANKLE SPRAINS</td><td>H</td><td>HIP PAIN</td><td>L</td><td>LIFTING FURNITURE</td><td>ONGOING PAIN</td></tr>
</table>

ONGOING PAIN

So, rather than banking on an injection or a couple core stability and strengthening exercises, which are common suggestions for treating a herniated disc, I'd recommend a combination of treatments. These include teaching Nancy to use the tonic muscles in her core and hips while using neurodynamic and fascial mobilizations to treat the fascial and nerve restrictions she developed. Dry needling and other techniques to reduce the myofascial trigger points in her back and hip would be necessary, as the trigger points could be their own source of pain. We would also have to address the scar tissue formation in her right ankle, since her limited dorsiflexion was the first of many injuries that accumulated to her pain. If we didn't treat it, she'd always have alterations in the way she walks and runs. All of these treatments would allow allowed her to improve her threshold line and, consequently, her activity line began falling below that line.

By applying this broad treatment regimen, as well as educating her on the exacerbating stress factor, Nancy found relief from the pain in her back and her right leg for the first time in more than ten years. She was shocked to learn that all the things she had done as an adolescent and as a student could have been the cause of unresolved pain that had lasted for so long. While she would have to continue learning how to correctly use the tonic muscles in her core and hip, maintain her ankle mobility, and be mindful of her stress levels, she was ultimately out of pain. She could once again go through life with an activity curve that stayed, for the most part, below her threshold line and gave her more bandwidth to live.

Nancy's case is a classic example of a peripherally sensitized back injury that should be seen in the context of her history and not just as a single lifting injury. My hope is that her Movement Story gives you a better idea of how something that seems like one injury is actually just the straw that broke the camel's back. If you think about your pain in the same context, is there a moment you might have lifted something awkwardly or did something randomly that caused an intense pain or injury? Rather than assuming it came out of the blue, can you see how it might be the culmination of other incidents?

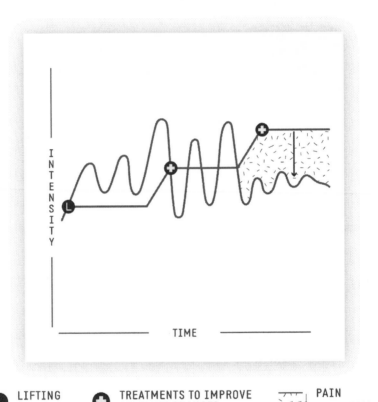

LIFTING FURNITURE

TREATMENTS TO IMPROVE REMNANT CHANGES

PAIN REDUCTION

TREATMENTS TO IMPROVE REMNANT CHANGES / PAIN REDUCTION

Understanding that your body is highly connected and that your pain is more likely an accumulation of previous episodes rather than an isolated occurrence, gives you the tools to find and fix the source (or sources) of your pain. Keep this in mind as we move forward, and ask yourself:

• Are there any places in my body where I might have remnant changes from previous injuries or pain?

• Can I think of a health practitioner who would understand the remnant changes I might be experiencing?

In the next section, we'll explore some of the more significant changes that don't necessarily occur in the joints, muscles, or fascia, but rather have the potential to affect the systems that process pain itself.

Changes that Affect Pain Itself

When it comes to pain, we've only scratched the surface on the subject. We've alluded to the fact that you can experience different types of pain, and, so far, we've discussed two types: peripheral sensitization and peripheral neurogenic sensitization. Peripheral sensitization is the typical pain you expect to experience. This is what you feel when you cut yourself with a knife or sprain your wrist and it hurts. We also talked about peripheral neurogenic sensitization, which is when nerves become sensitized, causing symptoms like numbness, tingling, and burning in your arms and legs. But there are other types of pain that can cause unresolved pain. The three most common types include: central sensitization, autonomic pain, and affective pain.

Central Sensitization

Central sensitization differs from peripheral sensitization in that the signal to the brain comes from receptors within your spinal cord versus the nociceptor cells outside your spinal cord. According to the Institute for Chronic Pain, "Central sensitization is a condition of the nervous system that is associated with the development and maintenance of chronic pain. When central sensitization occurs, the nervous system goes through a process called wind-up and gets regulated in a persistent state of high reactivity. This persistent, or regulated, state of reactivity lowers the threshold for what causes pain and subsequently comes to maintain pain even after the initial injury might have healed."[19]

Central sensitization starts at your spinal cord, where the nerves that extend to your legs and arms lead back to your spine. In the example of the ankle sprain, the sensitization would involve the lower back lumbar nerve roots. In this area, a structure called the dorsal root ganglion (DRG) lies on the back corner of both the left and right sides of your spinal cord. Here, the DRG essentially acts as a train station that accepts, receives, and transmits sensory signals from all over the body including increased nociceptive impulses, temperatures, touch, and vibrations.

Because the DRG is connected to so many other sensory fibers, it can become overly stimulated, inflamed, or sensitized. When that happens, it can lower your pain threshold much faster than a typical injury can. So instead of having a simple ankle sprain, or even mild back pain, the DRG perceives pain in response to sensations like light touch, cold, heat or vibration. In the worst cases, it may become reactive to even light or sound. All of these stimuli from outside your body can influence the nerves that send messages to the DRG in your spine, making a sensitized area that gets irritated easily and relays incessant messages of pain to your brain.

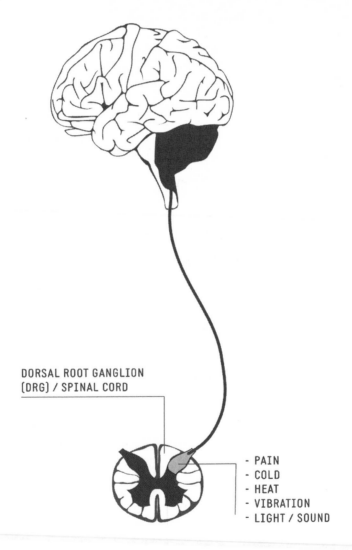

DORSAL ROOT GANGLION
(DRG) / SPINAL CORD

- PAIN
- COLD
- HEAT
- VIBRATION
- LIGHT / SOUND

For someone dealing with central sensitization, it may be difficult to pinpoint the source of the pain. They might have described their experience to health practitioners only to feel crazy. How could an ankle sprain possibly lead to light or sound or heat sensitivity? But what's really taking place is the DRG in your spinal cord has gone haywire; it can no longer tell which signals are causing problems and which are standard stimuli.

Because of the variety of sensory receptors that converge at the DRG, the brain cannot decipher what sensation is causing the pain. Now light touch, loud sounds, hot showers, or cold weather can exacerbate your pain, likely leaving you feeling confused and frustrated. The good news is this: regardless of which method your body uses to control pain—peripheral sensitization or central sensitization—you are not crazy, and you are not alone. Your pain, whatever form it takes, is real, and, more importantly, it can be treated. However, treatment strategies that address central sensitization issues are more focused on making changes at the spinal cord and central nervous system level, and not just what is on the periphery of your body where you feel pain that many of the remnant changes we have discussed fit with peripheral sensitizing pains. I recommend finding a physical therapist that is qualified to assess and treat central pain issues, as many may not feel comfortable doing so.

Autonomic-Related Pain

As I've mentioned, your body has another type of nervous system known as the autonomic nervous system. The autonomic nervous system is comprised of two main sub-systems: the sympathetic and parasympathetic nervous systems. The sympathetic nervous system controls your fight-or-flight response, while your parasympathetic nervous system is responsible for calming you down. In an ideal situation, your body will utilize one system or the other depending upon whether you need to be engaged or relaxed.[20]

However, many times your sympathetic nervous system takes over and goes into overdrive. People who are highly driven and run on adrenaline, for example, typically fuel themselves with their sympathetic system. Stress, anxiety, performance, achievement, laser focus—for them, it's all systems go all the time.

What most people don't know is that a significant portion of your autonomic nervous system is housed both in your brain and along your spine. There are nervous system structures that reside just outside the vertebrae of your spine, in your mid back or thoracic spine. These structures are called the autonomic ganglia, or the sympathetic ganglia, more specifically.

The autonomic ganglia are the nerve cells that control your sympathetic response. The more they're engaged, the more active your fight-or-flight response will be. In addition, your autonomic ganglia are directly linked to the neural connections of your internal organs. If you experience stress and upset stomach at the same time, it's because the autonomic nervous system reacts and sends signals to your gut when you're stressed, making your gut more sensitive or irritable. In fact, acid reflux, gastric issues, and bowel issues might all be related to an overactive sympathetic nervous system.

Or, if you've been diagnosed with an internal organ condition, such as colitis, your thoracic nerve roots and autonomic ganglia may have become sensitized as well. This happens when the inflammation in your internal organs sends inflammatory signals back up the nervous system, called retrograde impulses. There are many cases like this, when we see patients who have a problem with their internal organs, like acid reflux, and also have pain or hypersensitivity in their mid-back as a result of sensitization.

We refer to these sensations as autonomically or sympathetically maintained pain.[21,22] It's not surprising then that pain that occurs simultaneously may be connected, and on a more drastic level, sympathetically maintained pain can manifest itself in your extremities as well as your core. One of the most extreme cases of this type of sympathetically maintained pain is a syndrome known as Complex Regional Pain Syndrome (CRPS). Although there are different types of CRPS, CRPS is generally seen as a complex problem that can present with severe symptoms, including extreme pain, swelling, color change in the skin, and sensitivity to touch.

In many cases, patients have difficulty even putting weight on the affected area, and the sensitization of the autonomic nervous system is a primary driver in how CRPS develops and sustains. If you think you might experience CRPS or some form of autonomic related symptoms, realize that treatment strategies are more complex and will require a team of qualified health practitioners that understand its nature. Similar to central sensitization, you should find a physical therapist and other health practitioners and ask if they have the skill set to address central and autonomic pain-related issues.

Affective-Related Pain

Affective pain essentially refers to the emotional or mental component of your health, also known as your affect, and its contribution to your unresolved pain. For example, if you feel anxious or depressed because your pain won't let you do the things you enjoy, your affect may be a result of your pain; however, sometimes your affect can be the driving force behind why you're experiencing pain.[23]

While I'm not a clinical psychologist, psychiatrist, or mental health counselor, I have a long history of dealing with patients who suffer from unresolved pain issues. The beauty of doing what I do as a physical therapist is that I'm frequently able to understand a person's affect from a different perspective. Although many people shy away from seeing a mental health counselor because they're not fully aware of the depth of its impact, or they choose to avoid it, physical pain can be a different motivator. If pain limits their lifestyle, they may be forced to see a physical therapist to get moving again. Since they're coming to see me for a physical pain, patients are often unaware something affect-related might be influencing them.

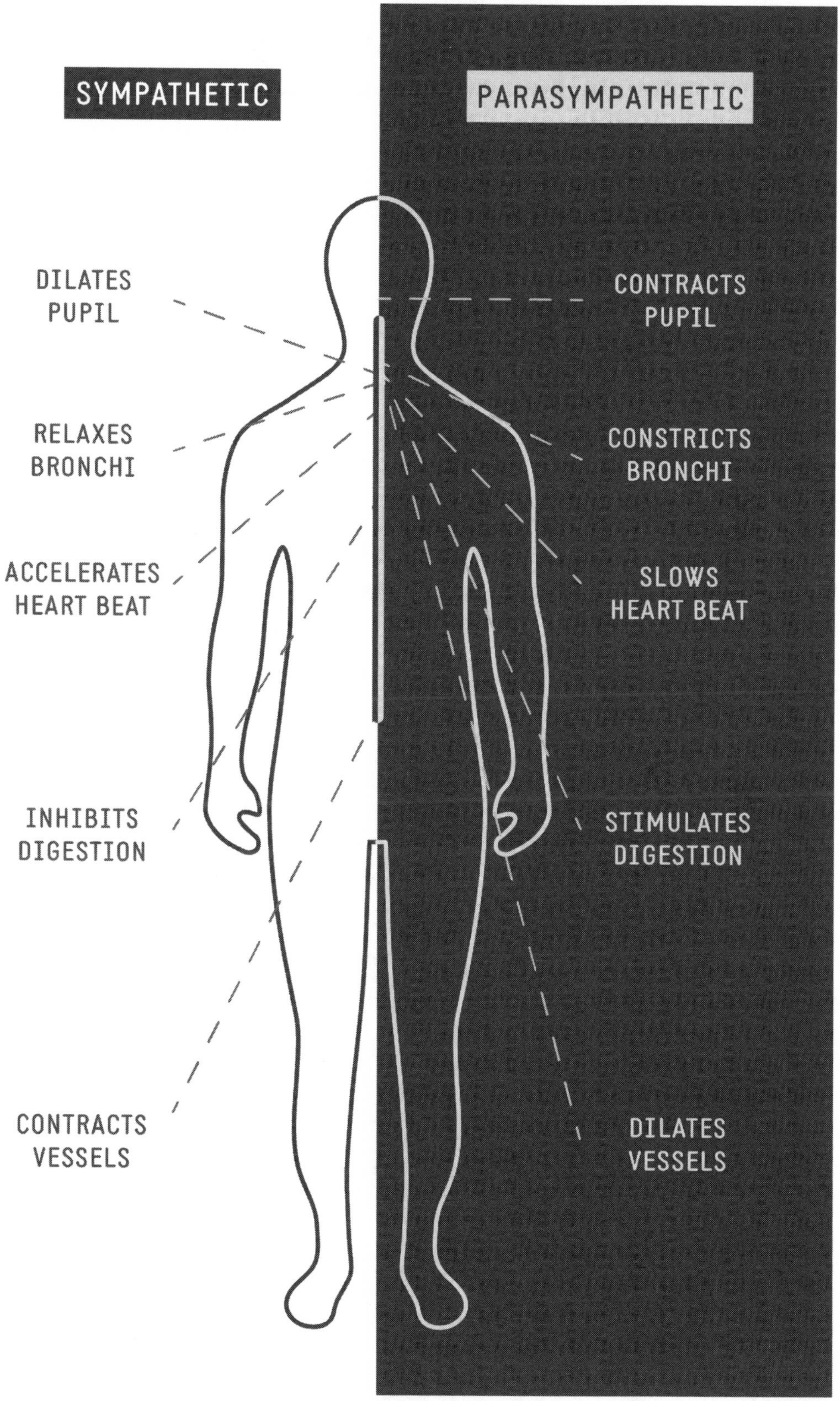

SYMPATHETIC

PARASYMPATHETIC

DILATES
PUPIL

CONTRACTS
PUPIL

RELAXES
BRONCHI

CONSTRICTS
BRONCHI

ACCELERATES
HEART BEAT

SLOWS
HEART BEAT

INHIBITS
DIGESTION

STIMULATES
DIGESTION

CONTRACTS
VESSELS

DILATES
VESSELS

Through an assessment and evaluation of the patient, I can explore not only the physical reasons behind their pain, but I can also discover their story through the Movement Story process. This way we uncover the root causes within the patient's own belief system, which may fuel the fire that led them to pain and maintained their unresolved pain state.

Motivating Factors and Belief Systems

In my experience, when someone is confronted with a pain that stops them from doing the things they want, they essentially have two choices: either try to push through the pain or avoid it like the plague.

A Toughen-up Attitude

Do you remember the story of Ben that was mentioned earlier in this book? He worked out and exercised obsessively because deep down he was afraid of having cardiac issues like his father, who died young. It wasn't until Ben realized his innate fear of meeting the same fate as his father did he come to grips that he was pushing his own body to the point of physical breakdown. And that motivation would never go away until he found peace and learned that exercising in moderation would be just as effective in optimizing both his cardiac and physical health. Only then was I able to help Ben take control of the physical injuries and pain he was experiencing.

Example: The High-Intensity Interval Training (HIIT) Junkie

A similar type of patient I commonly see are those who are attracted to the world of high-intensity interval training (HIIT). It has largely appealed to those looking to maximize their workout time by exercising in intervals that work different areas of the body by mixing cardio, flexibility, and strength in a short timeframe. Usually they even have modules set up that let you compete against your class or an internet platform that lets you compare yourself to others.

For this example, we'll talk about someone named Heather. Now forty years old, she decided to start running with a group of friends to get in shape when she was just seventeen. At that point she didn't realize how much she would love running! It was quick, practical, and social. Overall, it was a great workout, and Heather loved it so much she ran four or five times a week as an outlet for stress. She quickly began to chase a runner's high, or an addiction to the endorphin release she got by pushing herself harder in stride and distance.

By the time she hit forty, Heather had found other means of exercise to release endorphins. She became heavily involved in classes at Orange Theory Fitness, a group fitness gym that uses heart-rate monitors while participants work out in different ways. During the class, participants are encouraged to track and maintain a target heart rate, in the orange zone, which is the recommended range for good cardiac health while exercising. The class also shares a scoreboard showing performance, so participants can see how well they're doing within the class.

Orange Theory is a great way to train. Their trainers are aware of certain cardiac issues that enable them to provide guidance around when to progress and when to hold back. It's ideal for those who need a target to aim for along with guidance from the instructors, and Orange Theory attracts people like Heather, who was ultimately a competitor. She didn't necessarily need to compete against other people, but she always challenged herself. Forward progress was the goal; she thought she could always do better and rest was for the weak.

But at the age of forty, which was an aging milestone in her own mind, a pain in her left hip flared to the point where it hurt to run, take the stairs, or even sit down. Of course, she didn't rest. She took it upon herself and just kept running through it, telling herself to toughen up! "I'll get through this," she'd swear. "I'm not going to let turning forty be a sign of old age!"

Heather's case is important for two reasons. The first is that, while it may not be exactly the same case, many of us continue to push through pain and hope it will go away, only to find it getting worse. Second, how effective would it be for a physician or physical therapist to treat Heather's hip pain through injections, exercises, or other means, without also addressing her value system? Managing her addiction to the runner's high is just as important to treating her pain so she can safely return to the sports and workouts she loves.

It's another example of how health practitioners can become too myopic in treating a specific joint or muscle without examining the context of the patient's story. We need to consider what motivates the patient to injure herself. If the person cannot figure it out themselves, then it's the responsibility of the health practitioner to help them understand the danger as well as provide measures to address the issue.

The Avoid-it Mentality

Contrary to the ultra-aggressive personalities who try to push through their pain, there are also people who choose to simply avoid the activities that cause them pain. In some cases, that can be a good strategy, as there are people who should not put themselves in harm's way; however, they may develop such a fear of injury that they end up avoiding any activity that *might* cause them pain. This belief system, known as a fear-avoidance model, can be tricky because while it may not seem like a problem, a person can become overly risk averse.

For this example, we'll use a woman I treated named Sheri. She had sustained whiplash in a car accident that left her with chronic neck pain. For some reason, her neck pain wouldn't go away, and she eventually developed sharp, debilitating headaches. To make it worse, her job as a hairstylist required her to stand for ten-hour workdays, cutting hair in the salon. This may not sound like much strain on someone's neck, but after holding her arms up all day long to style her clients' hair, Sheri found that her profession only worsened her neck and shoulder pain. After work, her neck pain would be so sharp she would race home just to lay down.

Even before the car accident caused her neck pain, Sheri had already begun to hate working as a hairstylist. Her parents were both celebrity hairstylists, famous to movie stars and the wealthy, and expected her to carry the torch. But she always felt she was called to do something more independent; something she could call her own and not be in her parents' footsteps. She wasn't thrilled by being known as 'little Sheri' or known to just live off her parents' notoriety.

As her neck pain worsened throughout her workday at the studio, she started to hate her job even more. She found herself calling in sick or making excuses to leave early. She stopped asserting herself in her job and her parents were disgruntled about her performance and the reputation she was unable to uphold. Eventually she started resenting her parents because she felt they forced her into a profession she didn't enjoy, and she began to avoid driving out of fear of getting into another accident. It didn't help that her neck pain was only getting worse.

Sheri is an example of how pain can heighten, or serve as a catalyst to, one's underlying stresses or emotions. It can trigger decisions that may seem rational, but are ultimately fueled by anxiety or depression. It can also lead one to altogether avoiding certain things that were never major issues or even elements of a normal, daily routine. This fear-avoidance behavior can spiral into other behaviors and actions that cause more distress, alter relationships, and impact everyday life. But with unresolved pain that keeps getting worse, and a set-in belief system, we can sort of understand why Sheri would want to avoid her pain as much as possible.

Yet, just as with Heather, health practitioners cannot simply treat Sheri's neck pain and exclusively blame the car accident for its persistence. Without addressing her entire thought process, what she believes, and how it impacts her life, the practitioner won't be able to fully address her unresolved pain. Injections and exercises may help partially or temporarily, but addressing the tissue and structural changes that occurred in the accident *and* considering the effect that drives her decisions is the only way to truly help Sheri heal.

Changes to the Brain: Neuroplasticity

It would be easy to say, "Hey, get a grip and change your mindset!" And sometimes people just need a wake-up call to see their behavior from another perspective. When that happens, the prognosis is usually better and resolution is much quicker; however, sometimes a patient needs more than a Come-to-Jesus talk. Because as people start to foster these deep-rooted belief systems, there are actually physiological changes that occur within your brain. These changes reset and rewire different neural conduction patterns, changing the way the brain functions, perceives, believes, and makes decisions about how we move and live.[24]

This concept is called neuroplasticity, which is defined as the "capacity of neurons and neural networks in the brain to change their connections and behavior in response to new information, sensory stimulation, development, damage, or dysfunction."[25]

Think of an electrical circuit that has certain wiring designed to allow a light switch to turn on a light. If the wiring is reworked, the signals won't conduct as well or power any switches. This is essentially what neuroplasticity can do to you—it can alter your decision-making ability and your belief system based on previous occurrences or beliefs that had been ingrained in your brain through trauma, repetition, and other reasons.

Unlike a tight muscle, it's not easy to stretch your brain and get it working again. And while I'll be the first to say I'm not an expert in neuroplasticity, it's important that you're aware of how your affect can influence more than your beliefs; it can also physiologically remap the way your brain works. Fortunately, there are a multitude of inter-disciplinary interventions designed to improve neuroplastic changes, like medications, counseling, and electrical stimulation. Yet, as with most interventions, treatment needs to be coordinated between qualified health practitioners to be effective.

Summarizing Remnant Changes

Remember that everything we've covered regarding the different types of remnant changes your body can experience is an overview. Also, what I've shared about the possibilities of central sensitization, autonomic symptoms, and affective components only scratch the surface when it comes to the level of research and clinical work being devoted to unresolved pain. However, if you can relate to any of the areas we just discussed, I encourage you to reflect on how they may affect your Movement Story and the differing types of pain or injuries you may have incurred. I invite you to also consider what your MSG looks like, based on your changing thresholds to pain caused by the remnant changes you have developed, or your increased sensitivity, whether it be peripheral, neural or central sensitization, or any autonomic or affective factors that may be involved.

Of course, not everyone will have neuroplastic changes or mood-altering pain behavior. My goal is simply to bring it to light so you can make sense of your situation and the symptoms you're experiencing, and I hope it has broadened your perspective on what you might be going through. If you think they apply to you, it would still be best to consult with a practitioner who has had formal training in these areas.

NOTES

_____

_____

_____

_____

_____

_____

_____

_____

KEY POINTS TO REMEMBER:

- **No pain does not mean you are normal again**: Just because the experience of pain may go away after you are injured does not mean that things go back to normal.

- **Small changes. Big effects**: There are several remnant changes that may occur in your body that can either maintain your pain or lead to compensations that can lower your threshold and cause further injuries later.

- **Pain can change**: Pain itself can also alter, causing heightened responses through central sensitization, the autonomic nervous system, and neuroplasticity.

Section 2.2:

Evaluate Your Body's Design

Assessing Your Body's Design

Now that you have your pain narrative and you understand how initial and remnant changes contribute to your pain, it's time for you to learn how you can assess your own body, how it moves, and how it functions. Based on your pain narrative and what you know so far about how your body works with unresolved pain, we'll use the next section to explore specific details about how your body may not be as efficient, symmetrical, or level as it should be. You might start to notice differences in the way you stand, walk, bend, squat, or perform other movements that pertain to your life.

As you identify these things, know that there may be some steps you can take on your own to immediately address any imbalances; however, you'll most likely need to seek the help of a qualified health practitioner to deal with some of the more complicated asymmetries. Please know that not all physical therapists will see the things you might observe, and it's important you work with someone who listens to you and acknowledges your concerns so they can provide more detail in helping you.

Here are the four areas of your body we'll assess in this section:

- Posture;
- Textural Observations;
- Functional Movement; and
- Sport- or Activity-Specific Movements.

Posture

The first thing to consider is the hard structure of your body, or what we'll call posture. Usually physical therapists can determine a lot simply from the way you stand or walk. At different angles, standing postures alone can reveal essential information that you yourself may be unaware of.

Looking at your body from a hard structure standpoint can help identify more extreme outliers that may have a major impact on how the body works. You can tell whether one leg is longer than the other, whether your spine curves abnormally, how low or high the arches of your feet are, for example. Before we move forward, though, it's important for you to know that finding imbalances like these does not necessarily mean you'll be in pain forever. It will simply influence your treatment strategies.

Before we start the assessment of your posture, I'd recommend you wear minimal or fitted clothing during your evaluation. It's important that you're able to see your body easily and accurately. Now, look at yourself in a mirror, from every possible angle. Without judgement, just take notices of some of your body's obvious landmarks. Where it's applicable, try to compare the symmetry and <u>proportion</u> between your right and left sides. Then, ask yourself the following questions at every angle as we go, and don't forget to take notes! Noticeable imbalances may be hiding some valuable information about your ongoing pain. Let's get started.

From face on:

1. Are my shoulders the same height? Does one look higher or lower than the other?

2. Does my waistline look level? Is one side higher or lower than the other?

3. What about my feet? Are they flat? Are my arches high? Is one flatter or higher than the other? Does one turn inward or outward more than the other?

As you examined your body, what did you find? Were there some nuances? An imperfection here and there? Notable imbalances? For some people, these imbalances won't have any effect on their lives. And while your body may never be perfectly symmetrical, when it comes to your pain, these asymmetries could point to less obvious aspects of your pain story.

For your body to work most efficiently, the goal is to make its foundation as balanced as possible, and most imbalances can be treated through physical therapy techniques that improve the overall symmetry and efficiency of your body. For now, just do your best to take note of any indicators that stand out in your body.

CORRECT
FUNCTIONAL
ALIGNMENT

DYSFUNCTIONAL
ALIGNMENT

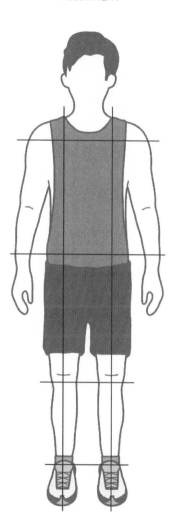
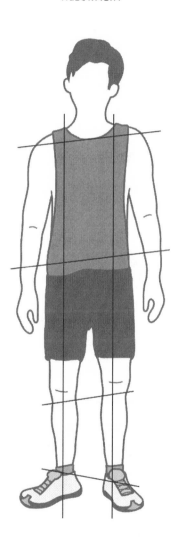

Textural Observations

Just as we examined the hard structure or posture of your body, we'll also look closely at the quality of your body's composition. This is less about noticing areas where you may have more fat, and more about looking qualitatively at how your body looks. The composition of certain areas of your body will tell us more about the health of your connective tissues.

Have you ever been surprised by how an acupuncturist can tell if you have an infection simply by looking at the color of your face? Well, it's common for pain and dysfunction in our internal bodies, whether organ- or musculoskeletal-related, to reveal themselves on the surface of our skin. That's why taking note of any textural observations across your body's tissues could give us more insight into your unresolved pain.

For our purposes, we'll evaluate seven tissue characteristics for potential pain implications, including:

1. Excessive bone growth;
2. Scar tissue;
3. Swelling;
4. Skin tone or color.

Again, with or without a mirror, examine your body for obvious landmarks, ask yourself the proposed questions, and take note of anything you notice. Ready? Here we go.

Excessive Bone Growth

When looking at your body, keep an eye out for any extraneous, bony shapes that stick out farther than usual. (This is not to be confused with a broken bone, which may protrude from your skin, too. If you have a broken bone, you should see a doctor immediately.)

The most common example of excessive bone growths that can contribute to ongoing pain is a bunion, or, medically, a bunion of the 1st metatarsophalangeal (MTP) joint. If you have a bunion, usually on the inside of your first toe's big knuckle, you'll see an extra bone growth extending inward, toward your other foot. Depending on how prominent your bunion is, it can be reddish in color, painful, or cause the big toe to bend outward, toward your second toe.

Where do bone growths come from? A well-established physiological principle known as Wolf's Law states, in layman's terms, that whenever repetitive or excessive force or friction is placed on a bone, the bone itself will start to grow extra bone in that area under pressure. It's your body's natural defense against sustained pressure; an attempt to fortify its structure so it can withstand the added force.

From a developmental perspective, bone growth is a perfectly normal process. Everything you do as a child—sitting, crawling, walking—helps your bones grow. To some extent, applying force and weight to your bones is actually required to develop their strength; however, applying extraneous force to your bones for long periods of time can cause them to keep growing unnecessarily, creating bone growths.

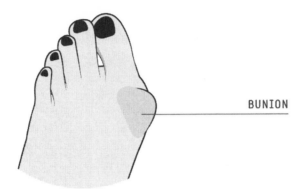

BUNION

If you have a bunion, or another notable bone growth, it's a good indication that your body is compensating for an imbalance somewhere. What starts as a minor issue may ultimately lead to pain in other parts of your body, as extraneous force in one place is carried throughout the nearby tissues, muscles, and joints needed to perform a function. A single bunion, for example, can cause your knee to turn inward or your hip to lose stability. Therefore, it's important to not write off a little bone growth, as it can be a signal of inefficiencies that contribute to your greater Movement Story.

Scar Tissue

Scar tissue, as we've discussed, can largely impact your mobility. Having a limited range of motion can influence how the rest of your body moves, so it's important your scarring isn't overlooked. Once again, with or without a mirror, examine the skin around your body. Keep an eye out for old scars, either from surgeries, fractures, or other major traumas.

While you can disregard small, superficial scars like skin abrasions or minor procedures, remember that some scarring (like with the ankle sprain) may not show up externally. As such, there are two perspectives to consider when it comes to your scar tissue. One is locally, or at the area immediately surrounding your scar, and the second is in the areas connected to the scar site, where scar tissue can affect other parts of your body.

Starting with the local scar sites, examine any obvious scarring on your body. If you've had surgery, like an ACL reconstruction or a knee replacement, you may have a vertical line down the front of your knee cap. Let's use this as an example of how scar tissue can impact the rest of your body. If you didn't have the scar, your skin, the connective tissues underneath it, and your muscles would be flexible and permeable enough to handle different stresses and motions.

Even if your physical therapist helped you regain almost all your range of motion, your knee's ability to fully bend or extend will still be limited compared to your other leg. This happens mostly because scar tissue is less elastic than your normal skin tissue, and it changes in relation to the proximity and size of the incision.

If scar tissue limits your ability to fully move the joint around it, the joints above and below it will also be forced to work differently. The same is true for nearby muscles. If your muscles cannot flex or contract because of stiff scar tissue, the other corresponding muscles will adapt their motion as well. Over time, the limitations can set off an improper sequence of events that cause your other joints, muscles, ligaments, tendons, and nerves to respond differently. Just like a bone spur, scar tissue can contribute to more of your Movement Story than you might think.

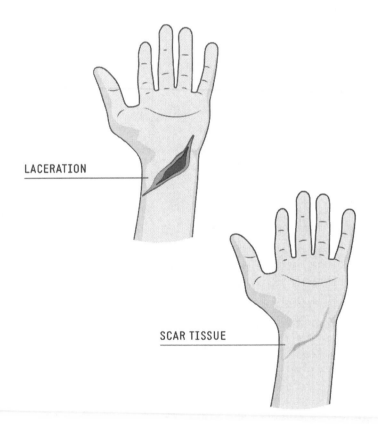

LACERATION

SCAR TISSUE

Swelling

Next, examine your body for any swelling. Do you notice residual or ongoing swelling anywhere? More specifically, is there one joint or area in particular that's still swollen from a surgery or injury? In most cases, ongoing swelling is an indication that your body is detecting tissue or joint dysfunction that hasn't fully healed or continues to be aggravated.

Knees and ankles tend to be very typical locations for low-grade swelling. Even if it isn't painful, swelling can be a sign of infection. As we discussed, it's part of your body's natural defense system, meaning that ongoing swelling can point to soft tissue trauma. Take note of anything that looks larger than normal and include it in your Movement Story overview.

Skin Tone or Color

Your skin, which is essentially just another connective tissue like your muscles or ligaments, can also tell you secrets about your pain. As you evaluate your body's characteristics, look out for areas near your pain site where the skin itself looks abnormal. Does it look or feel different from the rest of your skin? Is it glossy or sensitive to touch?

If that's the case, it can indicate inflammation of sensory nerves in your body. Changes in color, like a reddish hue, are more common signs of an inflammatory state. Whereas pale areas can be a result of limited blood flow, and blue-tinted areas can be caused by a lack of <u>vascular return</u>, or the flow of blood from the periphery back to the right atrium. In addition to inflammation, these colorations may imply a medical pathology that warrants further exploration and should be included in your Movement Story.

Summarizing Textural Observations

Before we move on to the next section, take time to write your observations:

- List any significant textural observations that stood out

- Note two or three observations you think could be factors in your unresolved pain

NOTES

_____

_____

_____

_____

_____

_____

Functional Movement

As a physical therapist, I can usually determine the source of a patient's pain simply by watching them move. In this section, we'll go through a series of movements that will let you do the same. In order to understand the complete manner in which your body works, it's important to observe yourself and the quality of your movements. But to keep it simple, we'll go through three basic movements you can do that will give you a significant amount of information about the efficiency and fluidity of your body. They include your:

- Gait;
- Squat; and
- Arm Raise.

Gait

The first thing to observe is the way you walk. For this you'll need to find a mirror with some room to walk in front of it. Then walk toward the mirror and watch the way your legs move, the way your arms swing, and the way your torso moves. As you do this, ask yourself the following questions:

Looking at your legs, ask yourself:

1. Do my feet generally point forward? Does one point outward or inward?

2. Do my knees look like they are moving straight forward, pointing toward the same direction in which I'm going? Or is one turned outward or inward compared to the other?

Looking at your arms and your torso:

1. Do my arms swing back and forth equally as my legs swing? Or does one arm swing less or drop down more than the other?

Be aware that any sense of asymmetry is likely to contribute to your pain. Additionally, this exercise is a good way to see the physical manifestations of any remnant changes that might exist within your connective tissues. If your ankle is stiff from scar tissue formation, for example, you'll probably notice that ankle and its foot point outward more than your other ankle. You might also notice that your heel comes off the ground sooner than the other heel, as you probably push off the ball of your foot earlier.

Meanwhile those with an inhibited gluteal or butt muscle might see their waistline drop or sway as they walk. This movement indicates your gluteal muscles aren't contracting enough to hold your leg and pelvis up properly, and as a result your pelvis or waistline isn't perfectly stabilized. You may even see compensations above and below your hip, like your knee turning inward or your opposite shoulder dropping down, as you step through with the leg on your inhibited side.

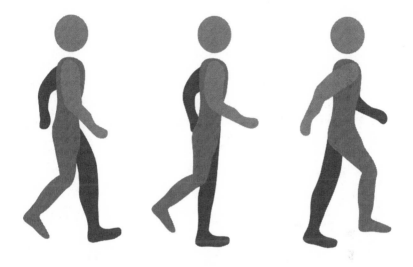

Squat

If you cannot see how your body might adapt or compensate while walking, you may see it by squatting, as this movement requires more mobility and strength. If your knees can handle it, stand in front of the mirror and watch your body as you squat down. Ask yourself:

1. Do both knees bend in line, facing relatively forward? Does one knee turn inward or outward more than the other?

2. Does one heel lift off the ground or does one foot twist outward more than the other?

If you're able, and if you want to learn more about your squat capacity, do a partial squat on one leg and see if you notice any other asymmetries or qualitative imbalances. Just like the way you walk, any areas of your body that don't line up as we'd expect can indicate that your pain may be a result of the different changes your body has gone through following pain or injury.

OBSERVING YOUR SQUAT

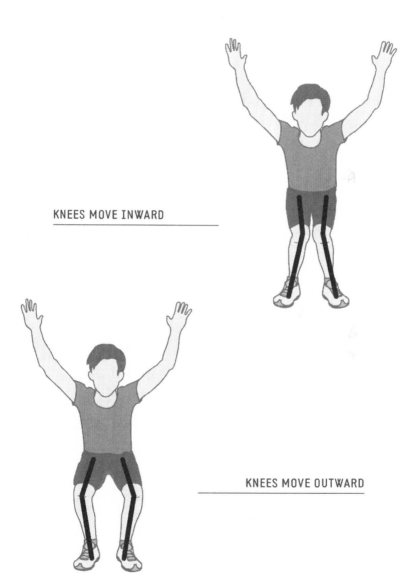

KNEES MOVE INWARD

KNEES MOVE OUTWARD

Arm Raise

Changes in movement patterns can also be seen in the upper body. One way to examine this area is to simply observe how your arms raise over your head. Looking at the mirror face-on, raise both arms out sideways and then up over your head. Ask yourself:

1. Do both of my arms raise to an equal height? Is one higher than the other?

2. If they're even, does one elbow stick out to the side or the front more than the other?

Just as there's a certain order to the way you walk, there's also a certain order and fluidity to the way your arms raise over your head. If you have pain in your hand, elbow, shoulder, or neck, you'll probably find that the injured side looks different from the other when you raise your arm.

Most commonly it is the shoulder blades, or scapular muscles, that are inhibited. These will work like your gluteal muscles in your leg. That means they're designed to establish the foundation for how your arm moves in space, and if those muscles don't work properly, you'll likely see your upper shoulder, or upper trapezius muscles, working harder to compensate. As such, you may be able to see your trapezius hike up as you lift your arm.

POOR
ALIGNMENT

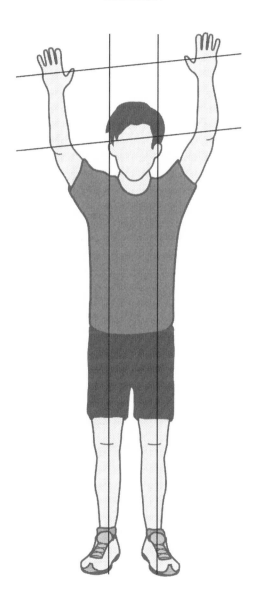

Functional Movement and Your Body's Design

As we move back toward the idea of your Movement Story uniting your narrative pain story and your body's physical design, it's important to understand how everything works together. In the section that discussed Your Body's Design, we talked about the different kinds of remnants that can occur after an injury. These can include muscle inhibition, scar tissue, myofascial trigger points, fascial and nerve restrictions, and even changes in your motor control and movement patterns. Now consider how common functional movements, such as the way you walk, squat, and raise your arms, can reveal how the different inefficiencies of your body have accumulated.

You see, if you have scar tissue in your knee that wasn't treated properly, how well do you think the functional movement of your squat will be? What if you had a herniated disc in your neck that caused radiating nerve symptoms down your arm, and now you try to repeatedly raise your arm to serve in tennis or paint a ceiling? What happens if, in addition to causing you pain, the significant myofascial trigger points that developed in your calf also reduced the mobility of the muscle, limiting your ability to extend through your foot and ankle?

After twenty years of practicing, I'm still fascinated by how the human body can adapt to all the different dysfunctions or restrictions it may have. Even though it can be an imperfect vehicle at times, more often than not, it adapts to keep going. The problem is that once we begin testing our body's bandwidth, we eventually end up pushing past our threshold time and again. And while the pain often subsides, letting you return to your routine, this time you feel stuck with your unresolved pain.

But I wrote this book to help you see the whole story, so you can understand all the physical changes that can follow the first time you sprained your ankle as a teenager, why having underlying body image issues fuels you to compete at a high level, or why being born with a structural abnormality can be the catalyst for how your movement patterns function today. I believe that the more you understand how your body works, both physically and emotionally, as well as how you've learned to adapt and survive, the more likely you'll be to address those issues.

Summarizing Functional Movement

Now that you've taken note of your posture, your textural observations, and your functional movements, you should have a better idea of the quality of your movements. But before we move on to the next section, take time to write your observations:

- List two or three things that stood out as you observed your functional movement.

- Note how you think they might contribute to your unresolved pain.

NOTES

_____

_____

_____

_____

_____

_____

_____

_____

Effects of Over-Specialization of Youth Sports and Performing Arts

For those who were highly committed in playing a specific sport or performing art as you grew up, you may find that your basic functional movement patterns reveal how your body adapted to playing those sports or arts. For example, I played competitive tennis as a child through high school. I had an advantage playing tennis, as I am left-handed. The spin on my serve was opposite of what was normally expected from a usual right-handed opponent, so it would throw them off from hitting my return of serve effectively. My coach would have me repeatedly work on my serve to make sure it was one of the main weapons in my game. However, there were many times, after playing weekend tournaments and long enduring matches, that my left shoulder would ache; sometimes I would feel sharp pain that could even be debilitating. If you know the serving motion in tennis, you know that it requires much power and rotation in the shoulder to generate a lot of spin and speed on the ball. That force on my shoulder made my shoulder muscles not only tired, but it also started developing myofascial trigger points, fascial restrictions, and even shoulder joint structural changes in the ligaments and joint capsule.

Not knowing then how repetitive motions like the tennis serve can cause that much wear and tear on my shoulder, I am now left with a shoulder that is not as mobile as my right one. On a basic functional movement arm raise, my left arm is unable to raise as high as my right. There is a lot of muscle tone around the shoulder muscles, and the joint simply does not rotate as well as the other one does. This is a manifestation of the different remnant changes that developed in my shoulder from playing years of tennis—and they persist to this day, even though I rarely play tennis anymore.

Treatments such as dry needling work to improve my fascia and myofascial trigger points surrounding my shoulder. This helps improve my overall joint mechanics in my shoulder, but there will always be less mobility in my left shoulder due to the amount of playing I did when I was younger. This decrease in mobility can affect me in other normal activities, like painting a ceiling or throwing my kids in the air when we're in the pool, because my inability to properly raise my arm can put more stress on my shoulder or on surrounding joints, such as my neck or back. Thankfully I know what my arm can handle, but if you're not aware of your limitations, you are left wondering why your shoulder or neck goes out on you with one lifting/throwing episode.

It's similar to the case with Nancy and all the adaptive changes her leg went through by playing soccer at a high level. That become an improper foundation for her leg to give her the correct support, and when she lifted the furniture, her back was injured because it was compensating for the lack of leg mechanics she developed from previous injuries.

My example of the developmental changes in my left shoulder can be easily discovered in other sports, performing arts, or repetitive activities we have done, especially when we were younger and our bodies were growing, changing, and shaping. In many cases, these adaptive changes can be at the cornerstone of why you structurally have unresolved pain issues.

Here is another example: youth who play sports or engage in performing arts that require a lot of extension or backwards arch in their mid and lower back, overtime, develop a hyperflexible spine. Their joints, ligaments, and muscles all stretch out to allow the gymnast the picturesque pose as they stick their landing, the ballet dancer to gracefully extend backwards to hold their positions, or the volleyball player to arch their back as they jump in the air to reach their shoulder and cock it back to spike the ball. Those who excelled in any of these activities were usually the best because they could get in that ideal position that creates optimal power or movement needed for that sport or performing art.

But although they are no longer playing at that type of level, their back is severely and highly extended, and it shows in simple, everyday postures, like standing or sitting. Now working a desk job, taking care of kids, or just doing daily chores like gardening, they are the people who find the 'average Joe' type of things to be extremely difficult. They are also often the ones with a 'push-harder' type of mentality, so when it hurts to do something, they tend to just grin and push through, only to eventually be debilitated by some random pain.

So as you go through the basic observations of your postures, textural observations, and functional movements, do not be surprised to see something that may be reflective of those sports or performing arts you so highly devoted yourself to when you were younger. Try to piece together the different remnant changes that you may have developed from those activities and injuries that may have occurred during those times. Combine them, and you might find the first key in understanding why you have had persisting pain for years. It also gives you some direction on areas you need to improve to get back to life.

Summarizing Youth Sports and Performing Arts Over-Specialization

As with the rest of your assessment, take time to write down your observations before we move on to the next section:

- What changes in posture, textural observations or functional movements do I see in my Body's Design due to the sports or performing arts that I participated in when I was younger?

- How do I think these factors contribute to my unresolved pain, and what are some strategies or interventions that I might implement to improve these changes I have incurred from my previous sports or performing arts activities?

NOTES

_____

_____

_____

_____

_____

Revisiting Your Movement Story

In the first half of this book, we worked together to establish your own narrative that spells out all the cascading events that accumulated to cause your unresolved pains. So far in this half, we made sense of how these events impact the specific way your body is designed to function. By now we know that when pain and injury occur, changes take place in your body and it finds a way to compensate so that you can keep moving through life. My hope is that by describing and listing your pain complaints, how they worsen, and the unique things about yourself, you've been able to see your pain in a new light.

Then, if you've been playing along, you also took time to take a closer look at yourself in a mirror. Not necessarily to question your existence or judge your appearance, but to get a good, objective look at your posture and the way you walk, bend, and squat. You should have also examined the textural context of your body, looking at swelling, discoloration, or excessive tone. You took note of ways you and your body might be using to protect yourself from further injury, and you reflected on all the small things you did to push yourself further. Perhaps now you can see how all these things became the foundation for an injury that, after enough time, repetition, or a traumatic event, propelled you into a state of unresolved pain.

Together, all of that information forms your Movement Story that lays out your entire history of activity, the ways you tried to raise your bar or threshold, and how much or how little bandwidth you have when it comes to physical and emotional capacity.

Because your Movement Story is unique, let's talk specifically about your Story using the knowledge you have now about how your body works, how it handles pain, how remnant changes accumulate, and how your brain can adapt.

Even if you can picture your graph in your head, it may be helpful to draw the details of your Movement Story so it makes perfect sense. Remember that the x-line is a relative reference of time that could represent your entire life or could be a short window during which time your pain began creeping in and became ongoing. It could represent the time you were training for a marathon and you tracked your distance, cadence, and time. Whatever time it spans, make the time span relative to who you are. Then map the two lines that depict your graph: your threshold line and your activity curve.

For your Threshold Line, think about where your line started in the first place. This is usually the place where you decided to commit yourself to a new activity, sport, or workload. Think about how many times you tried and managed to raise the bar by working and training harder. Then think about the moments when your threshold line may have dropped. Think about the time you broke an ankle and formed scar tissue, limiting the capacity of your leg to squat efficiently. Or the time you herniated a disc in your neck and developed inflammation that restricted the nerve, decreased its elasticity, and caused burning symptoms in your right arm. That might have decreased the threshold of your arm so that when you reached for your purse or briefcase in the backseat of your car, you felt a sharp pain in your shoulder.

For your Activity Curve, pick a time in your life when you were relatively pain-free. At this point, your activity curve should be much lower than your threshold line, because your body is not experiencing pain and has significant room, or bandwidth, to handle more load and more stress. Now think about the time your activity curve finally hit your threshold line and stayed above it, indicating that you entered the form of unresolved pain you're experiencing now. That moment could have been a trauma like a car accident or lifting a heavy box. It could have been a sports injury or a repetitive injury like painting your ceiling. Or it could be the moment you suddenly woke up with unceasing pain and had no idea what caused it.

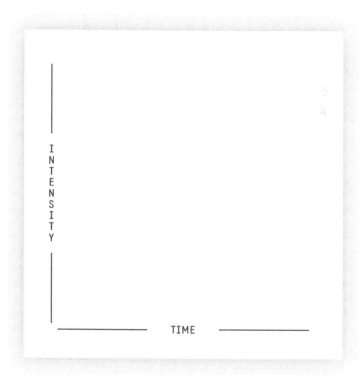

More importantly, see if you can make some connections between the beginning of your activity curve, where there's a lot of bandwidth, and where you are now with your unresolved pain. Think about all the different activities you've done that may have led up to this point. Perhaps there were times you sprained your ankle and felt a sharp pain that went away with rest. In this case, your activity curve might spike above your threshold line, indicating the distinct pain you experienced, only to drop below it once again. But, as inflammation and scar tissue caused remnant changes, your threshold line would still slightly decrease and your activity curve would not go quite as low as it did before. However minimal, your graph should show less bandwidth or capacity than before you sprained your ankle.

Once you've marked significant points, start adding in the other parts of your narrative story. Think about any injuries you may have sustained in sports, the time you threw out your back lifting something, or the years sitting too long to work or study caused your neck pain to flare up. Even if that pain went away, think about what it looks like in terms of your activity curve and how it may have changed your threshold line.

When you've finished your Movement Story Graph, I hope you'll see how all the previous injuries, physical or emotional stressors, and traumas you might have endured led to an eventual tipping point in what your body could handle, finally leaving you in the state of pain that lingers above your threshold line and doesn't come down.

This is the big picture I want you to understand: that there are a handful of variables and factors that are involved. Because there are no identical stories, there is no one-size-fits-all protocol for healing. You have to take your entire story, the remnant changes you may have, and the types of pain you may be experiencing (peripheral, central, neurogenic sensitizations and autonomic or affective pain) to understand all that may be contributing to your pain.

I realize it can be a daunting task to track your entire history on a linear map. Even the best clinicians have a hard time doing it. But remember that pinpoint accuracy isn't necessary. The point of the exercise is to conceptualize your own Movement Story by plotting incidents that may not seem important alone, but together show the relationship between your injuries and your unresolved pain that you may have been missing. Like the George Seurat paintings, your Movement Story should show the grand scheme of your unresolved pain so that perhaps your clinicians can see it too.

When you finally see the big picture of your unresolved pain, you have that AHA! moment, and you can find some peace of mind, comfort, and hope. In fact, simply understanding your entire Movement Story may bring enough peace to calm any anxiety you have about the unknown, that you might even experience a reduction in pain because your fight-or-flight system can finally come out of overdrive. You may start acknowledging how some of your own mindsets and affective components contribute to your pain, and realize how changing your perspective can allow the endorphins to kick in and encourage relief.

It's also possible you'll feel a little overwhelmed by all the information, and that's OK. My hope is that you at least have some more nuggets of information that you can take with you to your doctor, therapist, or other health practitioner so you can ask more questions about how they may contribute to your pain. Hopefully you find a practitioner who can help you see how it all fits together, finally make sense of why you have unresolved pain, and share solutions that address your entire Movement Story.

But even after all your hard work, the greatest challenge remains: how do you get yourself out of this unresolved pain state? It's not an easy task. Once your pain takes off and you develop central sensitization, autonomic pain, or affective types of pain that create anxiety, depression, or hopelessness, it may seem impossible to simply find an exercise that fixes it all. Now it becomes a process to which you need to commit yourself and stay focused. That's why I want you to have the tools to make sense of what might feel like madness, and I hope mapping your Movement Story gave you at least some comfort in that regard.

With that, the next logical question is, what now? How do you treat this and get rid of your unresolved pain? In the next section, I'll share some practical ways you can start on the right path, and I'll make recommendations for the team of health practitioners you should seek to continue moving forward on your journey. However, please know that I won't simply give five steps to fix your back. This book is intended for those who are determined to get to the root of their pain and are inquisitive enough to take ownership of their story so they can take the necessary action and make the commitment to heal.

Hopefully you've finally arrived at the point where you have enough understanding and depth of knowledge to draw your own Movement Story, and you now have a personal story and a physiological explanation of your pain. Now you're ready to take the next steps toward finally resolving your pain.

KEY POINTS TO REMEMBER:

- **Movement is a diagnosis**: There are some practical ways to observe how your body moves, and these ways can demonstrate the types of pain and injuries you may experience.

- **Movement is medicine**: Your observations can give you clues to how to start addressing things that can help resolve your pain.

SECTION 2.3:

Steps To Redefine Your Movement Story

This final section is designed to give you guidance on how to reduce your pain and begin to regain your life. Hopefully, by now, this book has helped you define your own Movement Story to better understand the root causes of your pain. Now you are probably thinking, "OK, I get why my pain is there, so how do I fix it?"

I wish there were one magic pill, exercise or intervention that would be the cure-all solution. But by now you have learned that there's no quick-fix. Instead, there are generally three main phases that you will need to progress through to not only get out of pain, but to ultimately enjoy your active life again. The three phases are:

1. Cutting the Edge off Your Pain

2. Getting Hold of Your Movement Story

3. Moving Forwards and Thriving

Cutting the Edge off Your Pain

When patients usually come to see me the first time, their symptoms are at their worst. This is because they are not only experiencing a lot of pain, but they also have no idea why it is really happening. This potentially is even after trying different medications, injections, surgeries, and other conservative treatments, such as massage, chiropractic, physical therapy, and acupuncture. Perhaps you can relate to the frustration of getting some short-term relief by any of the aforementioned solutions, but not seeing the pain calm down. At this stage of your unresolved pain, you are probably going a bit stir-crazy just to find some relief.

In this phase your goal is to simply get help and identify what is making the pain worse so you can experience some sense of reprieve. Again, as there is really no fix-it-all solution, your first step in uncovering pain relief options is to really understand your own unique Movement Story and define the factors that reveal your pain's behaviors. After all, if you don't quite know how something behaves, then how can you determine ways to correct it?

Essentially, our main goal in this phase is to stop your activity curve of your MSG from fluttering out of control and start decreasing it so that it may drop back down to the threshold line, thereby indicating that your pain intensity is becoming more manageable.

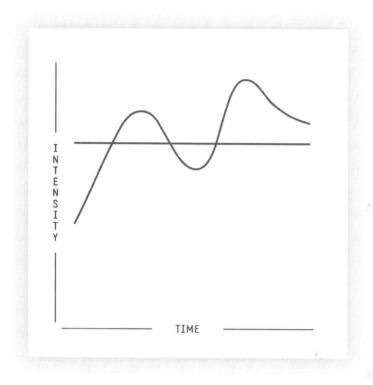

Now, look back and reflect on the pain narrative you discovered about yourself. Make sure you recall what your primary pain complaint was. Remember, also, how you thought your pain came about, through what we called your mechanism of injury.

From there, look back at the section that helped you 'Understand Your Pain Patterns.' In that section we helped you uncover three main areas known as your aggravating factors, easing factors, and

24-hour patterns that constitute how your pain behaves during the morning, afternoon, and sleep. It is within these areas that we can help you figure out how to cut the edge off the intense pain you are experiencing.

So, what are the things that really aggravate your pain?

I ask that question because most people focus solely on how much their pain hurts or how much it limits them from doing what they want to do. Instead, to find ways to calm your pain, you will have to identify any specific activities that really exacerbate your symptoms. In addition, you will have to determine what parameters make your pain worse. This can be based on duration or an intensity level, like how fast or how long or how hard you are trying to achieve your activity.

For example, people in acute or intense pain will often say that it hurts just to stand for ten minutes. Or, they may say, 'It hurts all the time, but especially when I pull weeds in my backyard for more than thirty minutes or when I start running after the first mile.'

So, rather than focusing on how much you hurt, hopefully you can identify those things in your life that provoke or aggravate your pain. If that is the case, you will first have to learn to limit the time or intensity of that aggravating activity, simply to avoid another spike in your activity curve that can send you into the intense, persisting pain that you may have grown accustomed to.

So, if it hurts to stand or sit for ten minutes, then I would recommend at this stage to only sit for five to seven minutes at a time. If running really hurts after the first mile, then I would say run a half or three-quarter mile and perhaps walk, so your pain does not shoot over the top. If gardening for thirty minutes aggravates you, then pull weeds for fifteen minutes and leave the deepest roots for someone else to do.

On paper all of that sounds like a no-brainer, right? But, in my clinical experience, I am amazed how often my patients need to be told to cut it back a bit with the goal to just cut the edge off their pain. As I mentioned before, I firmly believe the majority of us find ways to continue to achieve and get things done, even when we are in extreme pain. Perhaps you are able to still get your weeds pulled or sit in excruciating pain to get your office work done, but what good does that do in the long run? Not only are you experiencing more pain, but you are also causing more remnant changes that make you susceptible to injury and longer persisting pain. This is like someone pouring more lighter fluid on a bonfire that is already burning bright. The goal, in this first stage, is to just turn off that lighter fluid so we can attend to the bonfire.

Once I can get my patients to agree to cut things back, they will come back and commonly say, 'But yes, I've tried to rest and it may help a bit, but every time I try to run again or stand for more than ten minutes, my pain just comes back again...what's the point?'

My response to them is two-fold: One, at least they have found ways to cut the edge off their pain. Two, they won't get back to running or standing again without fully understanding what is causing that pain in the first place. From here, they need to continue to address those factors by looking farther into the pain narrative of their Movement Story that includes their easing factors as well as their 24-hour pattern.

EASING FACTORS

Looking back at your pain narrative, hopefully you were able to list at least one or two things that might be giving you a break from any searing pain you get during a normal day. Does sitting down for fifteen to twenty minutes give you at least some reprieve? Does laying on your back and taking a nap give your pain some relief? Do other interventions help? If so, use them! How about back braces or support devices, mechanical traction or modalities like electrical stimulation? Same thing. Wear them for the short term, just to cut the edge off your pain.

There is an entire industry based on gadgets, creams, or devices to give you pain relief. Perhaps they work for you, but regardless of their effects, I want you to focus on taking ownership of things you physically can do yourself to help ease your symptoms. If sitting down gives you a break from your pain because you are up on your feet all day long, then I would simply say that you should sit—not once you're in pain, but well before your pain intensifies. You may even have to take a sit break three or four times a day. It may stop you from running around all day long to get your checklist done, but at least you have less intense pain as the day goes on.

I know it may sound ridiculous to say a remedy to your pain is to simply take breaks, but again, you would be surprised to know how many patients in constant pain whom I treat will not simply stop and take a break, because they have to keep pushing through the day.

24-HOUR PATTERN

We discussed before how pain occurring at key moments of the day can reveal a lot about your pain behavior. If your pain is really intense first in the morning and loosens up as the day goes on, then you have a lot of inflammation. You will need to find ways to get your inflammation to calm down—medications, injections, and overall pacing strategies that do not provoke your inflammation are key at this stage.

If your pain increases as the day goes on and is triggered by what you do, then you need to focus on the things you are doing most of the day. As mentioned before, if you stand or sit all day long, then you might need to take more breaks. The goal for you is to simply make it to the end of the day with less searing pain, because pain that typically accrues as the day goes on is likely due to poor muscle control or other remnant changes that have developed in your body.

If your pain is most pronounced when you sleep, then you need to consider your sleeping positions. However, as I mentioned before, if you are feeling pain primarily at sleep and you have other compounding factors, such as weight loss or other medical conditions, then you need to see your physician to rule out any medical pathologies.

By looking more closely at your aggravating and easing factors, as well as your 24-hour pattern, hopefully you have been able to clarify the small nuances of how your pain behaves. From there, you can start to make small lifestyle changes, and, within one or two weeks, you will notice that your intensity of pain is not as extreme as it was. You will still be in pain, but perhaps it will be more tolerable, and maybe you'll even enjoy some pain-free moments.

If that is the case, your activity line on your MSG is declining and nearing your threshold line. Congratulations on meeting the goals of this first stage! Now you want to make changes that give you more long-lasting changes.

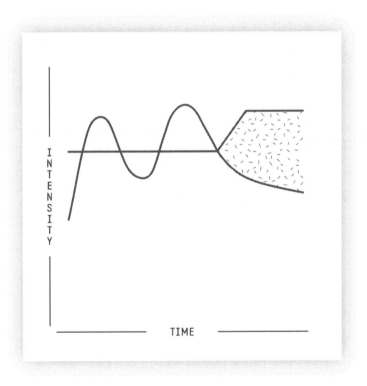

 NO PAIN / RAISING THRESHOLD / LOWER ACTIVITY

Getting Hold of Your Movement Story

Now that the edge of your pain has decreased, it's time to get a hold of it and start turning your Movement Story to your favor. So far, I have helped you find ways to get your activity curve to decrease and head towards, or just below, your threshold line. But, as you probably know already, resting and taking breaks will not be enough to get you out of pain in the long run. You also need to improve your threshold line that declined due to the adaptive or remnant changes your body has undergone through the years of your different injuries or pain episodes.

The goal in this second phase is to get your activity line and your threshold line to switch with each other, making your activity line below your threshold line. It is in these moments that you start to experience a real, longer lasting resolve of your pain.

So, how do we achieve this moment where pain no longer dominates your life?

Now it is time to make improvements to your body's construct as well, so that you can begin to restore its natural design. Look back and reflect on the key points in your observations of the different remnant changes that you may have; your posture, the way you walk, and the way you functionally move. Was there anything that really stood out to you? If so, can you make any correlation to why your pain is occurring? In addressing those things that may have a correlation to your pain, and improving them, will lead to a decrease in that pain, and you'll feel like you can move more freely.

For example, let's say you have chronic left knee pain. You have tried injections, medications, physical therapy, and even surgery, but it continues to hurt. In your pain narrative, you recognize you fractured your left big toe when you were much younger. When you then took the time to observe how your own body functions, you noticed when you walk, that your left foot turns out more than your right one and your left arch is flatter than your right as well. When you squat, you see that your left knee turns inwards more than your right one. You also notice that you have less muscle tone in your left buttock muscle.

In this example, hopefully by reading through this book, you understand your left knee pain is not necessarily the main issue. While it may be where your pain is located, your real problem stems from the lack of flexibility in your left first toe. It has affected the way you walk, and your body has compensated by turning your left foot out because your big toe is unable to bend the way it should to walk properly. The arch in your foot is beginning to flatten or collapse more because your foot has turned out. You also have less left hip strength because the way you now walk does not allow you to use your gluteal muscles the way they were designed. As a result, when you squat, your left knee starts to turn inwards because it does not have the proper mechanics from both above and below, since the hip and foot are not functioning properly.

So how do you begin to correct all that? If the above example is you, and you were my patient, I would aim to improve both your foot and toe mechanics as well as your left hip motor control. I would teach you to wear good shoes that help support your flattening arch. If there was room for improvement to increase the mobility of the left big toe, then I would teach you exercises, as well as perform hands-on techniques to improve that flexibility, as that is one of the major reasons your entire left leg is not functioning as well as it should. I would then aim to help improve the motor control of your left gluteal muscles that probably are laden with myofascial trigger points and have significant muscle inhibition.

As the foot and big toe improve in structure and function, you would notice that your left foot does not turn out as much and your big toe bends more, allowing your entire left leg to stay in the plane of motion it should when you walk.

As your hip strengthens by reducing the number of myofascial trigger points in your gluteal muscles, and the muscle is no longer inhibited, you will have the muscle control to walk and squat properly. When you squat, you would see a much less turn-in from your left knee. Not surprisingly, your left knee would hurt less because it is now moving in a more normal fashion with less stress on it as well.

Simple, right? From there, if you made the changes I mentioned before, not only would your pain decrease, but your threshold line and physical capacity to do things like squatting, walking, and going up and down stairs would improve.

You would have also learned, in the first phase, to cut your activities down—to not run or garden so much. During these activities that used to aggravate your knee, you would be attentive to your left leg mechanics to avoid your knee turning in as much.

In this scenario, your activity line is tailored and both your activity line and your threshold line would improve. And guess what? That ongoing pain in your left knee—that has left every health practitioner you've seen scratching their heads and wondering why your knee still hurts—starts to get some traction, and the pain episodes in your left knee lessen, to the point that you are able to do more without feeling the severe pain you once had.

This, of course, is a very simplified case, but it should lend insight on how to take steps to not only take back control of your pain, but to also enjoy some movement again. This approach of incorporating your entire Movement Story can be applied to essentially any pain in your body, matching it with your pain narrative while considering how your bodily movements have compensated.

This phase also may require a team of health practitioners to help you along the way. There are certain remnant changes that need the intervention of a physical therapist, chiropractor, physician, or other practitioner that can help reverse some of the physical changes in your body. However, it is still vital that you take ownership and understand how your own body and your own Movement Story work. You should not be dependent on someone else to fix things for you. Instead, you should have a stronger command and understanding of the things you need to take care of. In my experience, when you take responsibility for mitigating your pain, there is a much more lasting and impactful change.

Hopefully by now you have been able to take hold of the first two stages by cutting the edge off your pain followed by harnessing your Movement Story through correcting the adaptive changes your body previously made. If that is the case, then on your MSG, you are experiencing an activity curve that spends less time under the threshold line. With improvements in your threshold line as well, you are now experiencing more true pain relief. You notice you that can do a little more in your daily life without the acute exacerbations of pain that you once felt. What you are really experiencing is more bandwidth, or capacity, in your functional daily life that can withstand more stress, more load, and more activity without getting injured. If you have accomplished this stage, then congratulations once again! You are starting to overcome the pain that had altered your life for so long.

For most people dealing with ongoing pain, reaching the point of substantial pain relief and more activity might be enough. However, there is one more stage that I would encourage you to consider, and that is to see if you increase your threshold to the point that your own body can start to be more active and perform at higher levels without experiencing significant setbacks. Sure, you might be satisfied that you're out of major pain, but you are still susceptible to a resurgence of pain. That is because there still may not be enough bandwidth in your MSG to handle unexpected circumstances that can easily set you back. By aiming to raise your threshold line, your body has more resilience to withstand more. Your likelihood of recurrence of injury or pain drops, and you can enjoy an even more active life! Who wouldn't want that? If you do, then let's move on to the final stage.

Move Forwards And Thrive

As I mentioned before, I firmly believe that many of us have the innate desire to push our bodies. This could be in high-level sports or simply in sitting behind our computers for endless hours to ensure that our work gets done. Either way, it is natural to keep going—until something stops you. In this case, the deterring force is usually severe pain.

In the first two phases of restoring your Movement Story you not only have learned to cut the edge off your severe symptoms by understanding your pain narrative, but you have also learned to make physical changes to your body to improve the way it should work, so you can have more freedom of motion and a better threshold capacity. Now in this third stage, it is about learning to raise your threshold so your body can start achieving the things you desire to accomplish.

For example, nothing gets me more excited than helping a golfer dealing with a physical ailment that has not only affected their golf swing, but that has also compromised the power and distance behind their ball. When I explain to them that their golfing pain is caused by their narrative and changes in their functional movement, they initially get excited—they notice that, by making the necessary changes based on their Movement Story, their pain decreases. Moreover, using this approach, the golfer starts to improve the strength and flexibility that are critical for normal activities like squatting and raising arms overhead. Better yet, we also raise their threshold to have the sport-specific flexibility and strength necessary for the golf swing itself. This means that they are not only experiencing less pain, but they are now hitting the ball farther and straighter than they did even *before* they got hurt. Why is that? Because the golfer not only addressed their remnant changes that were hampering their basic fundamental movements, but they also made improvements in their body that were specific to the goals or activities they wanted to achieve.

In the example of the golfer, can we assume that just because someone is strong and flexible that they will hit the golf ball far? Golf requires highly specific flexibility and strength in certain parts of the body, and this flexibility and strength may be different than those found in someone who can do a deep squat. So, in order to have the most successful outcome, the golfer needs to train to optimize and achieve golf-specific movements. Once that is accomplished, the golfer will not only have less pain occurrences, but they will have a body that is specifically optimized for golf.

This example does not just pertain to golf. Whether you're a runner or a tennis player, or you practice another higher level sport or activity, you will need to train your body to have the capacity to handle the specific forces that are required in that activity.

This also pertains to the small daily things, such as sitting or standing for long periods of time, or gardening. Do you have the physical capacity in strength, motor control, and posture to stand all day long at a work conference? Do you have the capacity to spend twelve-hour days behind your computer to study for your exam or get your work project done, or stay in a half-bent position and pull weeds in your backyard?

No matter the activity, you will need to address the factors that are required to accomplish these specific activities. Yes, you may have overall good functional capacity to do most things, but in order to fully thrive in your life and prevent pain recurrences, you will need to optimize your body for these specific activities or goals.

This might be the fun—and perhaps more expensive—part. You may need to invest in a health practitioner or coach that knows the sport or activity in which you want to excel. That person you hire may be a golf performance trainer or a physical therapist that understands dancers' injuries. They will be aware of the specific nuances that the activity requires so you can maximize your body. You may also need to invest in equipment that helps you maximize your body's performance. You may need to invest in the best ergonomic chair for work so you have the best support to sit through those long days. You may need to find the best bike fitter that understands what bike frame and components fit best your body so you can excel on your mountain rides.

Again, your goal in this phase is to not only know your Movement Story and the pain factors from your past. You also need to take ownership so that you can raise your threshold line to allow your activity curve to go up without it spiking above the threshold line.

You will have more capacity to achieve the things you want to do and you will find more success in maximizing your body to be able to push it harder than you could before, with significantly less pain or injuries.

If you have been able to achieve all of this, job well done! Not only have you found ways to cut the edge off your persisting pain and made changes to get your daily life in order and less aggravating, but you are starting to thrive and live again as you enjoy the things you love.

So what happens if your pain flares up again? By now, in fully understanding your unique Movement Story, you should be able to quickly address the factors that have caused your pain and you should no longer have to withstand the duration of pain you once experienced.

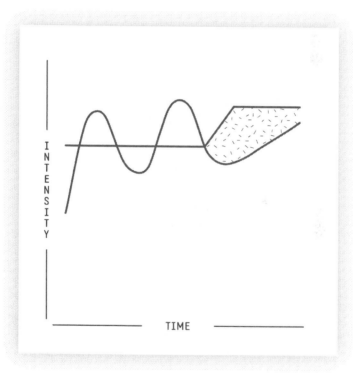

NO PAIN
ACTIVELY THRIVING AGAIN

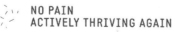

MSG: MOVE FORWARDS & THRIVE!

SUMMARY CONCLUSION

In conclusion, I hope this book has helped you look past your pain and appreciate the larger context, as it's portrayed in your Movement Story—the source of your unresolved pain. Hopefully by now you have gained enough insight to take ownership of your pain by making specific life changes to curtail your pain. More importantly, you can now start taking steps to live your life again. You should also have more knowledge in which health practitioners you should seek help from to get your body where you want it to go.

Everybody—and every body—is different, so it's impossible to have answers for each specific pain. This book was specifically designed to give you the broad construct with which to understand how your pain has manifested throughout your life.

However, in summary, here are the general steps that we have discussed throughout this book, and that you should take:

1. KNOW YOUR PAIN NARRATIVE

- Understand why your pain is unique to your personal story instead of focusing on what a single test or diagnosis says about your pain.

2. KNOW YOUR PAIN'S NATURE

- Identify the activities that both aggravate and ease your pain. This will give you an idea of how to keep your symptoms under control.

3. IDENTIFY YOUR REMNANT CHANGES

- Understand the specific remnant changes your body has accrued from previous injuries, surgeries, or your medical history.

4. OBSERVE YOUR BASIC MOVEMENT PATTERNS

- Identify any inefficiencies in basic movement patterns, such as the way you walk, squat or raise your arms overhead, and how these inefficiencies might reveal why your pain exists.

5. DRAW YOUR MOVEMENT STORY GRAPH

- Utilize the Movement Story Graph to draw a visual representation of how your pain has manifested.

6. MAKE CHANGES

- Start to make changes in your behaviors and activities to decrease the intensity of your pain.

7. SEEK HELP

- Find the right practitioners to help improve the remnant changes in your body so that your movement patterns and pain can be normalized.

8. REDEFINE YOUR MOVEMENT STORY

- Aim to improve your threshold and bandwidth so you have more capacity to perform and achieve without pain.

If you can get through these steps, then you should celebrate: you have overcome the chronic pain that has ruled your life for so long! With that, it's normal to have more specific questions that pertain to the pain that you might be experiencing. To help you further explore your own unique Movement Story, I have provided additional resources on my website, at www.BrianYee.com.

At the very least, my hope is that this book has empowered you to not only take control of your pain, but also take ownership of your own body; to reject being solely dependent on healthcare tests and interventions. Instead, I want you to feel like you are back in the driver's seat to live the life you aspire for—and your Movement Story that reflects it.

Definitions

Understanding the Terms that Relate to Your Body

Action potential: a spike in electrical activity caused when a neuron in your brain sends information down an axon, the long thread-like part of a nerve cell, to other cells.

Activity curve: the undulating line above the x-axis on your Movement Story Graph, which correlates the intensity of any activity over any amount of time.

Antegrade impulses: inflammation chemicals that travel from your spine into your arms, legs, hands, or feet.

Apical breathing: a process in which your body relies on muscles in the chest and neck for breathing, instead of using the diaphragm.

Ascending fibers: a nerve pathway that goes upward from the spinal cord toward the brain, carrying sensory information from the body to the brain.

Axon: the long thread-like part of a nerve cell used to transmit information to other cells.

Bandwidth: your ability to do an activity before reaching your threshold.

Central sensitization: the process in which sensory nerves in your spinal cord react to stimuli and send a pain signal to your brain.

Chemical mediators: chemical substances your body produces and sends to your nerves, muscles, or glands.

Clinical reasoning: The process by which physical therapists (and other clinicians) collect cues, process the information, come to an understanding of a patient's problem or situation, plan and implement interventions, evaluate outcomes, and reflect on and learn from the process.

Cortical pathway: a nerve system in your brain responsible for muscle and joint function.

Diaphragm: a dome-shaped, muscular partition that separates the thorax from the abdomen and assists with breathing.

Descending fibers: a nerve pathway that goes down the spinal cord and allows the brain to control movement of the body below the head.

Dorsal root ganglion: a cluster of neurons (a ganglion) located in the lumbar nerve roots.

Dorsiflex: the range of motion related to your ankle as it bends toward your shin.

Dry needling: a physical therapy technique practiced by inserting a dry needle, free of injections or medications, through the skin and into trigger points in the muscle.

Force closure: states that any external force applied inwardly helps provide extra support to the joints of the body.

Hip anteversion: a 15- to 20-degree inward turn of the hip socket.

Hip retroversion: a 15- to 20-degree outward turn of the hip socket.

Hip torsion: the rotational motion or rotational capacity of your hips.

Inflammation (or swelling): a physiological reaction caused by chemical mediators in your body to protect itself from further injury.

Inflammation mediators: see chemical mediators.

Inspired rib: a bodily formation that expands the lower rib cage as a result of sustained accessory breathing.

Movement Story: a unique approach to identifying the roots of your pain by evaluating both the integration of your pain narrative and your body's natural design.

Movement Story Graph (MSG): a visual representation of your body's everyday, physical abilities, where the axes, depicted by the x- and y-lines, represent time and intensity, respectively. The undulating line you see above the x-axis is your activity curve, and the horizontal line that rests above the activity curve and intersects the y-axis is your threshold line.

Muscle atrophy: a loss of mass in your muscle, specifically as a result of prolonged underuse.

Muscle inhibition: a shrinking in the cross-section size of the muscle due to a break in the connection to your cortical pathway.

Muscle tone: the size or shape of your muscle in its natural resting state.

Nerve guarding: your body's natural instinct to move in a way that protects or guards an inflamed or sensitized nerve.

Neurodynamics: the understanding of the relationship between the mechanics and physiology of your nervous system.

Neurotransmitters (or chemical mediators): chemical substances your body produces and sends to your nerves, muscles, or glands.

Neurogenic inflammation: inflammation along an entire nerve somewhere in the body.

Nociceptor: a special sensory neuron or fiber that receives inflammation mediators that then act as a gatekeeper of the way pain is generated and perceived, by sending warning signals to the spinal cord and the brain.

Peripheral sensitization: the process after an action potential occurs and the nociceptors send a signal from somewhere in your body (that is not considered part of your central nervous system) and up through your spinal cord, signaling your brain that something is wrong.

Proportion: the shape or size of one particular muscle compared to its opposing muscle.

Purpose: the reason for which something exists; its intended or desired result, aim, or goal.

Reciprocal gait pattern: the process in which your body uses its opposite sides in conjunction to keep you straight while you walk.

Scoliosis: a twist or curvature in the spine.

Sensory neuron: a neuron that is designed to receive and send information to your body or brain.

Symmetry: the correspondence in size, form, and arrangement of parts on opposite sides of a plane, line, or point; the balance between a muscle on one side of your body in relation to the same muscle on the other side.

Threshold line: the horizontal line that rests above the activity curve and intersects the y-axis, representing your bandwidth, or your body's capacity to handle any activity.

Trigger points: Sensitized areas within a muscle that can be a source of pain or contributing to different sources of pain and movement dysfunction.

Unity: the natural design of your bodily systems to function together, in a cohesive system.

Vascular return: the flow of blood from somewhere in your body back to the right atrium.

Wolf's Law: the principle that whenever repetitive or excessive force or friction is placed on a bone, the bone itself will start to grow extra bone in that area under pressure.

Endnotes

[1]   Andre Agassi, Open: An Autobiography. Vintage, 2010.

[2]   Blog entry: www.desiringgod.org/articles/injury-interrupted-my-idolatry

[3]   Butler DS & Moseley GL. Explain Pain. 2nd ed. Noigroup Publications: Adelaide, 2013

[4]   Mueller MJ, Maluf KS. *Tissue Adaptation to Physical Stress: A Proposed "Physical Stress Theory" to Guide Physical Therapist Practice, Education, and Research*, Physical Therapy, Vol 82, no. 4, p 383-403, April 2002.

[5]   How to Care for a Sprained Ankle." *How to Care for a Sprained Ankle*, The American Orthopaedic Foot & Ankle Society (AOFA, www.aofas.org/footcaremd/how-to/foot-injury/Pages/How%20to%20Care%20for%20a%20Sprained%20Ankle.aspx

[6]   "Donovan S, Brechter J, Sueki D. Tissue Injury and Healing. In: *Orthopedic Rehabilitation Clinical Advisor*. Marlyand Heights, MO: Mosby Elsevier; 2010.

[7]   Hides, J A, et al. "Evidence of Lumbar Multifidus Muscle Wasting Ipsilateral to Symptoms in Patients with Acute/Subacute Low Back Pain." *Current Neurology and Neuroscience Reports.*, U.S. National Library of Medicine, 15 Jan. 1994, www.ncbi.nlm.nih.gov/pubmed/8153825.

[8]   Miller, Jen A. "When the Diagnosis Is 'Dead Butt Syndrome'." The New York Times, The New York Times, 21 Dec. 2010, well.blogs.nytimes.com/2010/12/21/when-the-diagnosis-is-dead-butt-syndrome/.

[9]   Donnelly, Joseph M., and David G.. Simons. Travell, Simons & Simons' Myofascial Pain and Dysfunction: the Trigger Point Manual. Wolters Kluwer Health, 2019.

[10]   Shah JP, Gilliams EA. Uncovering the biochemical milieu of myofascial trigger points using in vivo microdialysis: an application of muscle pain concepts to myofascial pain syndrome. *J Bodyw Mov Ther.* 2008;12(4):371-384.

[11]   Shah, Jay P, and Elizabeth A Gilliams. "Uncovering the biochemical milieu of myofascial trigger points using in vivo microdialysis: An application of muscle pain concepts to myofascial pain syndrome." Elsevier, Journal of Bodywork and Movement Therapies, 8 Apr. 2008, drsvanderveen.info/PDF/Shah_Biological_milieu_of_MTP.pdf.

[12]   Shacklock, Michael. Clinical Neurodynamics: a New System of Musculoskeletal Treatment. Elsevier Butterworth Heinemann, 2015.

[13]   Stecco, Luigi, et al. Fascial Manipulation: Practical Part. Piccin, 2009.

[14]   Stecco, Luigi, et al. Fascial Manipulation: Practical Part. Piccin, 2009.

[15] Myers, Thomas W., et al. Anatomy Trains: Myofascial Meridians for Manual and Movement Therapists. Churchill Livingstone/Elsevier, 2017.

[16] Moseley GL, Butler DS. *Explain Pain Supercharged: The Clinician's Manual*. Adelaide City West, South Australia:NOI Group Publications 2017.

[17] Bergmark, Anders. "Stability of the Lumbar Spine." Acta Orthopaedica Scandinavica, vol. 60, no. sup230, 1989, pp. 1–54., doi:10.3109/17453678909154177.

[18] Page, Phillip, et al. *Assessment and Treatment of Muscle Imbalance: the Janda Approach*. Human Kinetics, 2014.

[19] Boivie J. Central Pain. In: Wall PD, Melzack R, eds. *Textbook of Pain*. 4th ed. Philadelphia, PA: Churchill Livingstone; 1999.

[20] Devor M, Seltzer Z. Pathophysiology of damaged nerves in relation to chronic pain. In: Wall PD, Melzack R, eds. *Textbook of Pain*. 4th ed. Philadelphia: Churchill Livingstone; 1999.

[21] Scadding JW. Complex regional pain syndrome. In: Wall PD, Melazack R, eds. *Textbook of Pain*. 4th ed. Philadelphia: Churchill Livingstone 1999.

[22] Moseley GL, Butler DS. *Explain Pain Supercharged: The Clinician's Manual*. Adelaide City West, South Australia:NOI Group Publications 2017.

[23]   Moseley GL, Butler DS. *Explain Pain Supercharged: The Clinician's Manual*. Adelaide City West, South Australia:NOI Group Publications 2017.

[24]   Moseley GL, Butler DS. *Explain Pain Supercharged: The Clinician's Manual*. Adelaide City West, South Australia:NOI Group Publications 2017.

[25]   Rugnetta, Michael. "Neuroplasticity." Encyclopædia Britannica, Encyclopædia Britannica, Inc., 28 Mar. 2019, www.britannica.com/science/neuroplasticity.

About the Author

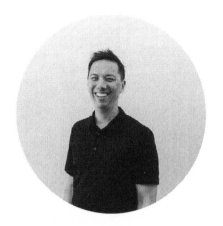

Dr. Brian Yee, PT, DPT is a Board-Certified Orthopaedic Clinical Specialist (OCS) and a Fellow of the American Academy of Orthopedic Manual Physical Therapists (FAAOMPT). A graduate of Northwestern University in physical therapy, Brian completed post-graduate physical therapy training at the University of Queensland in Australia and obtained his Doctorate of Physical Therapy from the Evidence in Motion Institute. He serves as Adjunct Clinical Assistant Professor at Mercer University Physical Therapy.

Brian has been published in the medical journal Spine, and was a contributor in the rehabilitation textbooks *Orthopedic Clinical Rehabilitation Advisor* (2010) and *Myofascial Pain and Dysfunction: The Trigger Point Manual* (2018).

He wrote *(Un)Resolved* to inspire others to take ownership of their body and of their pain, and to reassure them that there is a more comprehensive solution to pain than a test, diagnosis or intervention.

Originally from southern California, Brian now makes his life in Atlanta, Georgia, where he owns his private practice, Motion Stability Physical Therapy.

Visit www.BrianYee.com for more educational resources to help you understand your own Movement Story and to take the steps to live a pain-free and active life.

Made in the USA
Columbia, SC
28 April 2022

59543403R00155